AF364249

Practical
Pharmaceutical In-organic Chemistry
Second Edition

*Appended with Additional Experiments, Test for Purity and Assay
Methods of Indian Pharmacopoeia-2014 for Small Molecule Drugs*

Practical Pharmaceutical In-organic Chemistry

Second Edition

Appended with Additional Experiments, Test for Purity and Assay Methods of Indian Pharmacopoeia-2014 for Small Molecule Drugs

Bayya Subba Rao

M.Pharm., P.G. Diploma in Patent Laws (NALSAR), FAGE (MAN), Ph.D.,

Professor

V. Alagarsamy

M.Pharm., Ph.D.,

Professor & Principal

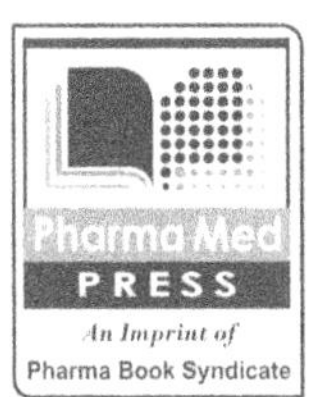

PharmaMed Press

An imprint of Pharma Book Syndicate

A unit of BSP Books Pvt. Ltd.

4-4-309/316, Giriraj Lane,
Sultan Bazar, Hyderabad - 500 095.

Practical Pharmaceutical In-organic Chemistry, *Second Edition by Bayya Subba Rao and V. Algarsamy*

Published by :

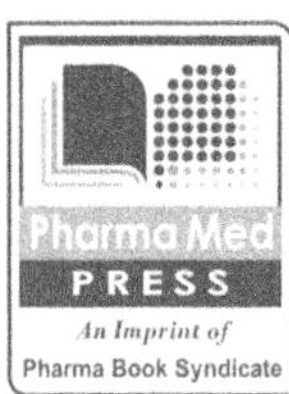

PharmaMed Press
An imprint of Pharma Book Syndicate
A unit of BSP Books Pvt. Ltd.
4-4-309/316, Giriraj Lane, Sultan Bazar, Hyderabad - 500 095.
Phone: 040-23445600, 23445688; Fax: 91+40-23445611
E-mail: info@pharmamedpress.com
www.pharmamedpress.com/pharmamedpress.net

ISBN : 978-93-86819-67-3 (Hardback)

Dedication

*This book is dedicated to
my father Late. Sri. Bayya Rama Mohana Rao,
my mother Smt. Bayya Lakshmi Kumari,
my wife, son, daughter, brother, sisters and all pharmacy fraternity.*

(Bayya Subba Rao)

Dedication

*This book is dedicated to
my parents, teachers and students*

(V. Alagarsamy)

Preface to Second Edition

A standard book is one which covers the concepts to the peak leaving apart the inclusion of the fundamentals. Such books are written by authors keeping in view the reader is well versed with the fundamental concepts. Indirectly, the author inculcates the habit of not only reading his book but also indulges the student to habituate to refer to other books for additional information and also get acquainted to other books. This is a part of making the student generate interest and quest for knowledge.

Once a stage has been reached, the student can understand any book by a single reading. A student should inculcate the habit of upgrading his standard but should not expect the book should come down to his standard.

Keeping in view of all in mind, the authors were putting all the efforts to generate initial level of interest by making a better understanding of the fundamentals. In the second edition, the authors made an attempt in putting efforts in inclusion of additional experiments that mimics several practical problems that arise while practicing the profession and inculcate the habit of identifying a problem and solving it logically.

The book covers with limit tests, synthesis of in-organic compounds used as drugs, a few procedures that ensure quality by conducting tests for purity, assay (quantitative analysis) of in-organic drugs, identification tests for anions, cations, separation of cations present in mixtures. Majority of the procedures are from Indian Pharmacopoeia, published by Government of India.

Special efforts were made in compiling all the assay methods used with respect to small molecules used as drugs as per Indian Pharmacopoeia 2014 and its Addendum published in 2015.

The book is a practical approach that also helps in quick reference during diploma, undergraduate, post-graduate curriculum not only relating to pharmacy profession but also helps for allied sciences who have relevant concepts.

The book is useful at Diploma, B. Pharm, M. Pharm, Pharm D, and Pharm D Post Baccalaureate education levels as well as informative while taking competitive examinations such as GPAT etc. In addition to this, the book is useful to the industry, researchers, teaching faculty, doctorates those who are new to the concepts.

The authors were told that several universities have deleted syllabus relating to in-organic drugs and such book will be useful for those graduates while practicing profession either at the industry, teaching or research levels. This is because, the inorganic drugs are still being used, available in Indian Pharmacopoeia and are available in the market.

Last but not the least; the authors would like to reveal that the current book is an outcome keeping in mind to impart fundamentals while taking care not to indulge the student into spoon feeding practices. Efforts were taken by the authors to include appropriate correct information and readers are requested to intimate the authors if any errors, deficiencies are identified so that necessary steps are taken for future upcoming editions.

- Authors

Acknowledgement

We take this opportunity in acknowledging our beloved students in their ample support for bringing this book.

Our sincere thanks to Dr. B. Suresh (President, Pharmacy Council of India, New Delhi), Dr. P. Gundu Rao (former Director, R&D, Divi's Laboratories Limited, Hyderabad), Dr. M. N. A Rao (General Manager, R&D, Divi's Laboratories Limited, Hyderabad), Dr. R. K. Goyal (Ex Vice-Chancellor, The MS University of Baroda, Baroda) for their moral support in bringing this book for the pharmacy students.

Our sincere thanks to our fellow colleagues in their support in bringing this book.

- Authors

Contents

3. Test for Purity

4. Assay

5. Identification of Anions and Cations

Anions

Cations

6. Semi-Micro Analysis

1

Limit Tests

Introduction

Impurity is defined as the presence of one substance in another substance in low concentration. Impurity can be an organic, in-organic, microbial, dust, moisture etc. In a pharmaceutical substance, the nature of impurity can be predicted provided we know the source through which it has been obtained. Impurities are imparted into the pharmaceutical substance through raw materials, intermediates, reagents, catalysts, solvents, reaction vessels, improper storage, cross-contamination, manufacturing errors, packing errors, microbial contamination, chemical instability, storage containers etc.

Water is a rich source for chlorides, sulphates, carbonates etc. Reactor materials used for manufacturing are rich source of steel, copper, iron, zinc, lead. Reagents, catalysts are rich sources of arsenic, antimony, heavy metals, lead, cadmium, mercury, which are potent nerve poisons on cumulative accumulation.

Hence presence of an impurity in a pharmaceutical substance may cause cumulative toxic effect, decreased therapeutic effect, change in physical and chemical properties, difficulty in formulation, in-compatibility, decrease in shelf-life, change in odour, colour, taste and appearance.

Since procuring pure pharmaceutical substance free from impurities is expensive and difficult process, Indian Pharmacopoeia, which is under the control of Ministry of Health & Family Welfare, Government of India provides permissible limit of a impurity and designate the pharmaceutical substance as standard provided it complies the tests given under individual monographs.

Limit tests are quantitative or semi-quantitative test designed to control small quantities of in-organic impurities, which are likely to be present in a pharmaceutical substance. Limit test for chlorides, sulphates, lead, iron, heavy metals and arsenic are official tests designed and mentioned in the individual monograph of pharmaceutical substance in Indian Pharmacopoeia.

The limit of impurity is provided in terms of parts per million (ppm $\equiv$ 1 μg $\equiv$ 10^{-6}g).

In these tests, standard opalescence/turbidity/colour/stain obtained by the reaction of known quantity of impurity with the reagent is compared with the test opalescence/turbidity/colour/stain obtained by the reaction of specified quantity of test sample (pharmaceutical substance) with the reagent. Hence limit tests are comparative tests in which both test and standard must be prepared simultaneously at the same conditions. The reagents used are dilute solutions so that the reaction is slow and sensitive. Additionally, the reagent selected should be less specific so that limits of several likely impurities can be accomplished.

In case of limit test for chlorides, sulphates, heavy metals and iron, Nessler cylinders are used for the test and the standard. Nessler cylinders are matched tubes of clear, colourless glass with a uniform internal diameter and a flat, transparent base. They are of transparent glass with a nominal capacity of 50 ml. The overall height is about 150 mm, the external height to the 50 ml mark, 110 to 124 mm, the thickness of the wall, 1.0 to 1.5 mm and the thickness of the base, 1.5 to 3.0 mm. The external height to the 50 ml mark of the cylinders used for a test must not vary by more than 1mm.

*Note***:**

(i)   Special alternations should be done while performing limit tests especially in case of insoluble and coloured pharmaceutical substances. In case of insoluble pharmaceutical substances (ex: activated charcoal), it is thoroughly extracted with boiling water and later the water is used for performing limit tests. In case of coloured pharmaceutical substances (ex: potassium permanganate), the colour is removed by chemical treatment like ethyl alcohol and later limit test is performed. One has to also remember that limit of impurity is fixed for individual pharmaceutical substance, but quantity of pharmaceutical substance to be tested for limit test is mentioned in individual monograph.

(ii)   Use directly the sample in case of liquid or in solution form as directed in monographs.

(iii)   If a test sample has to be made to fail in limit test for a particular impurity, add small quantity of standard impurity into the sample and perform the test.

(iv)   A turbid solution is a non-clear solution. Opalescence is a change in colour.

(v)   Select similar identical Nessler cylinders by keeping next to each other and the difference between 50 ml mark of both cylinders should not be more than 1 mm.

Diagram of Nessler Cylinders

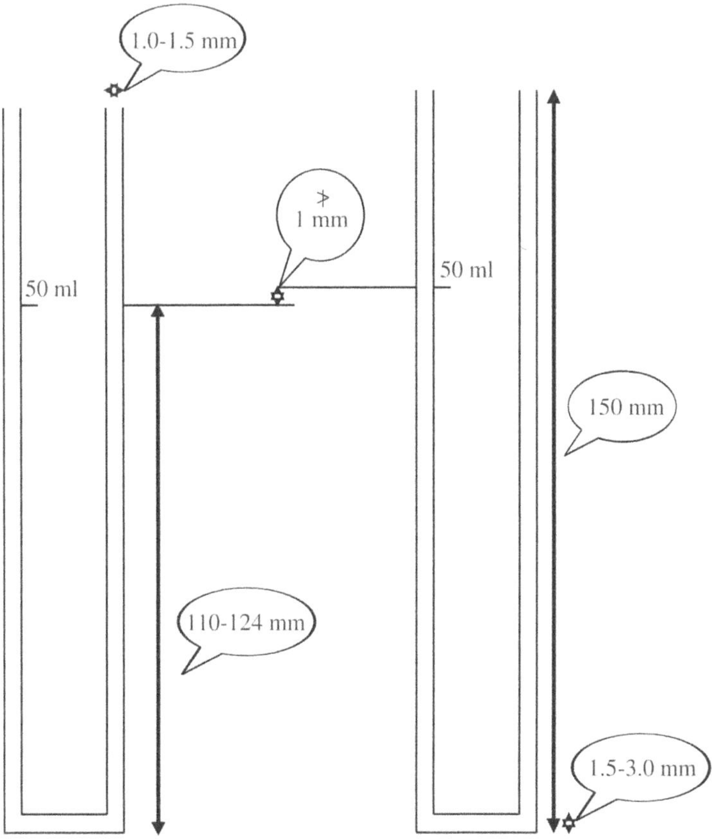

Experiment 01

Limit Test for Chlorides

Aim: To perform limit test for chlorides for the given sample.

Requirements: Nessler cylinders, glass rod, measuring cylinders, 1ml bulb pipette, 10 ml bulb pipette, dilute nitric acid, 0.1 M silver nitrate, chloride standard solution (25 ppm Cl), test sample.

Principle: In this experiment, the test opalescence obtained by the reaction of chloride impurities with silver nitrate is compared with standard opalescence obtained by the reaction of known quantity of chloride with silver nitrate. Dilute nitric acid is used to dissolve other impurities if present.

$$Cl^- \quad + \quad AgNO_3 \quad \xrightarrow{\text{Dil . HNO}_3} \quad AgCl \downarrow \quad + \quad NO_3^-$$
$$\text{opalescence}$$

The precipitate silver chloride formed is insoluble in dilute nitric acid and gives opalescence.

Procedure:

Test opalescence: Dissolve the given sample in 20 ml of water and transfer to a Nessler cylinder. Add 10 ml of dilute nitric acid, dilute to 50 ml with water. Add 1 ml of 0.1 M silver nitrate. Stir immediately with a glass rod and allow to stand for 5 minutes, protected from light. View transversely against a black background.

Standard opalescence: Transfer 10.0 ml of chloride standard solution (25 ppm Cl) into a Nessler cylinder and add 5 ml of water. Add 10 ml of dilute nitric acid, dilute to 50 ml with water. Add 1 ml of 0.1 M silver nitrate. Stir immediately with a glass rod and allow to stand for 5 minutes, protected from light. View transversely against a black background.

Test Solution	Standard Solution
Dissolve the given sample in 20 ml of water and transfer to a Nesseler's cylinder.	Transfer 10.0 ml of standard chloride solution (25 ppm) in to a Nesseler's cylinder and add 5 ml water.
Add 10 ml of dilute nitric acid, dilute to 50 ml with water.	Add 10 ml of dilute nitric acid, dilute to 50 ml with water.
Add 1 ml of 0.1 M silver nitrate solution.	Add 1 ml of 0.1 M silver nitrate solution.
Stir immediately with a glass rod and allowed to stand for 5 min, protected from light and viewed transversely against a black background.	Stir immediately with a glass rod and allowed to stand for 5 min, protected from light and viewed transversely against a black background.

Observation:

Test opalescence is not more intense than standard opalescence.

or

Test opalescence is more intense than standard opalescence.

Report/Result:

The given sample passes limit test for chlorides.

or

The given sample fails limit test for chlorides.

Preparation of Reagents:

1. *0.1 M silver nitrate:* Dissolve 17.0 g of silver Nitrate in sufficient water to 1000 ml. (Store in light-resistant containers)

2. *Chloride standard solution (25 ppm Cl):* Dilute 5 volumes of a 0.0824% w/v of sodium chloride to 100 volumes with water.

3. *Dilute nitric acid:* Contains approximately 10% w/w of HNO_3. Dilute 106 ml of nitric acid to 1000 ml with water.

Experiment 02

Limit Test for Sulphates

Aim: To perform limit test for sulphates for the given sample.

Requirements: Nessler cylinders, glass rod, 1ml bulb pipette, 2 ml graduate pipette, 5 M acetic acid, sulphate standard solution (10 ppm SO_4), test sample, barium chloride solution, ethanolic sulphate standard solution (10 ppm SO_4), 1ml graduate pipette.

Principle: In this experiment, the test opalescence/turbidity obtained by the reaction of sulphate impurities with barium chloride is compared with standard opalescence/turbidity obtained by the reaction of known quantity of sulphate with barium chloride.

Dilute acetic acid is used to dissolve other impurities if present.

$$SO_4^{2-} \ + \ BaCl_2 \ \xrightarrow{\text{Dil. acetic acid}} \ BaSO_4\downarrow \ + \ 2Cl^-$$
opalescence/turbidity

The precipitate barium sulphate formed is insoluble in dilute acetic acid and gives opalescence/turbidity. A known amount of potassium sulphate is added both in test and standard in order to increase sensitivity, rapid and complete precipitation by seeding. Ethyl alcohol is used to prevent super-saturation and thus producing uniform opalescence/turbidity. In the earlier editions of Indian pharmacopoeia, barium sulphate reagent containing barium sulphate and ethyl alcohol was used instead of ethanolic sulphate standard solution. Instead of acetic acid, hydrochloric acid was used. The change in the reagent does not effect the objective of the test.

Procedure:

Test opalescence: To 1.0 ml of a 25.0% w/v solution of barium chloride in a Nessler cylinder add 1.5 ml of ethanolic sulphate standard solution (10 ppm SO_4), mix and allow to stand for 1 minute. Dissolve the given sample in 15 ml of water and add 0.15 ml of 5M acetic acid, pour the solution in the Nessler cylinder. Add sufficient water to produce 50 ml, stir immediately with a glass rod and allow to stand for 5 minutes and viewed transversely against a black back ground.

Standard opalescence: To 1.0 ml of a 25.0% w/v solution of barium chloride in a Nessler cylinder add 1.5 ml of ethanolic sulphate standard solution (10 ppm SO$_4$), mix and allow to stand for 1 minute. Add 15 ml of sulphate standard solution (10 ppm SO$_4$) and 0.15 ml of 5 M acetic acid. Add sufficient water to produce 50 ml, stir immediately with a glass rod and allow to stand for 5 minutes and viewed transversely against a black back ground.

Test Solution	Standard Solution
Transfer 1.0 ml of a 25 % w/v solution of barium chloride in to Nessler's cylinder.	Transfer 1.0 ml of a 25 % w/v solution of barium chloride in to Nessler's cylinder.
Add 1.5 ml of ethanolic sulphate standard solution (10 ppm SO$_4$), mix and allowed to stand for 1 min.	Add 1.5 ml of ethanolic sulphate standard solution (10ppm SO$_4$), mix and allowed to stand for 1 min.
Dissolve the given sample in 15 ml of water and add 0.15 ml of 5 M acetic acid and pour the solution into a Nessler's cylinder.	Add 15 ml of standard sulphate solution (10 ppm SO$_4$) and 0.15 ml of 5 M acetic acid to the Nessler's cylinder.
Add sufficient water to make up 50ml.	Add sufficient water to make up 50ml.
Stir immediately with a glass rod and allowed to stand for 5 min and viewed transversely against a black background.	Stir immediately with a glass rod and allowed to stand for 5 min and viewed transversely against a black background.

Observation:

Test opalescence is not more intense than standard opalescence.

or

Test opalescence is more intense than standard opalescence.

Report/Result:

The given sample passes limit test for sulphates.

or

The given sample fails limit test for sulphates.

Preparation of Reagents:

1. *25% w/v barium chloride:* Dissolve 25.0 g of barium chloride in 100 ml water.

2. *5 M acetic acid:* Solution of any molarity xM may be prepared by diluting $57x$ ml ($60x$ g) of glacial acetic acid to 1000 ml with water.

3. *Ethanolic sulphate standard solution (10 ppm SO₄):* Dilute 1 volume of a 0.181% w/v solution of potassium sulphate in ethanol (30%) to 100 volumes with ethanol (30%).

4. *Sulphate standard solution (10 ppm SO₄):* Dilute 1 volume of a 0.181% w/v solution of potassium sulphate in distilled water to 100 volumes with the same solvent.

Experiment 03

Limit Test for Iron

Aim: To perform limit test for iron for the given sample.

Requirements: Nessler cylinder, 2ml bulb pipette, 20% w/v iron-free citric acid, thioglycollic acid, ammonia solution, iron standard solution (20 ppm Fe), glass rods, red-litmus paper.

Principle: In this experiment, the test colour (purple) obtained by the reaction of iron impurities with mercaptoacetic acid (thio glycollic acid) is compared with standard colour obtained by the reaction of known quantity of iron with mercaptoacetic acid.

Citric acid (iron-free) is used to complex metal cations other than iron if any present.

$$2\ Fe^{3+} + 2\ SH{\cdot}CH_2{\cdot}COOH \longrightarrow 2\ Fe^{2+} + HOOC{\cdot}CH_2{\cdot}S{\cdot}S{\cdot}CH_2{\cdot}COOH + 2\ H^{+}$$

$$Fe^{2+} + 2\ SH{\cdot}CH_2{\cdot}COOH \longrightarrow$$

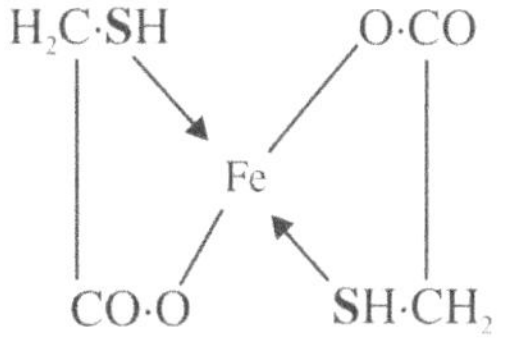

Ferrous Mercapto acetate/
Ferrous thioglycolate

In addition to forming complex with Fe^{2+}, thioglycollic acid acts as a reducing agent and converts Fe^{3+} to Fe^{2+} if any present.

The ferrous mercapto acetate formed gives purple colour in presence of citric acid. In addition to formation of metal complex other than iron, citric acid forms ammonium citrate buffer when ammonia is added to make alkaline, which in turn stablises the complex formed.

Procedure:

Test colour: Dissolve the given sample in 20 ml of water and transfer to a Nessler cylinder. Add 2 ml of a 20% w/v solution of iron-free citric acid and 0.1 ml of thioglycollic acid, mix, make alkaline with iron-free ammonia solution, dilute to 50 ml with water and allow to stand for 5 minutes and observe the colour transversely.

Standard colour: Transfer 2.0 ml of iron standard solution (20 ppm Fe) to a Nessler cylinder. Dilute with 20 ml water. Add 2 ml of a 20% w/v solution of iron-free citric acid and 0.1 ml of thioglycollic acid, mix, make alkaline with iron-free ammonia solution, dilute to 50 ml with water and allow to stand for 5 minutes and observe the colour transversely.

Test solution	Standard solution
Dissolve the given sample in 20 ml water and transfer into Nessler's cylinder.	Transfer 2.0 ml of iron standard solution (20 ppm Fe) to a Nessler's cylinder.
Add 2 ml of 20 % w/v of iron free citric acid.	Add 2 ml of 20 % w/v of iron free citric acid.
Add 0.1 ml of thioglycollic acid.	Add 0.1 ml of thioglycollic acid.
Then make the solution to alkaline with iron free ammonia solution.	Then make the solution to alkaline with iron free ammonia solution.
Dilute to 50 ml with water and allowed to stand for 5 min and observe the color transversely.	Dilute to 50 ml with water and allowed to stand for 5 min and observe the color transversely.

Observation:

Test colour is not more intense than standard colour.

or

Test colour is more intense than standard colour.

Report/Result:

The given sample passes limit test for iron.

or

The given sample fails limit test for iron.

Preparation of Reagents:

1. *0.05 M sulphuric acid:* Solutions of any molarity xM may be prepared by carefully adding $54x$ ml of sulphuric acid to an equal volume of water and diluting to 1000 ml with water.

2. *20% w/v iron-free citric acid:* Dissolve 20 g of iron-free citric acid in 100 ml water.

3. *Iron-free ammonia solution:* Contains approximately 10% w/w of NH_3 (iron-free). Dilute 425 ml of strong ammonia solution to 1000 ml.

4. *Iron standard solution (20 ppm Fe):* Dilute 1 volume of a 0.1726% w/v solution of ferric ammonium sulphate in 0.05 M sulphuric acid to 10 volumes with water. Contains iron in ferric state.

Experiment 04

Limit Test for Heavy Metals

Aim: To perform limit test for heavy metals for the given sample.

Requirements: Nessler cylinders, 1ml bulb pipette, dilute acetic acid, dilute ammonia solution, hydrogen sulphide solution, pH paper: 3-4 range, lead standard solution (20 ppm Pb), glass rods.

Principle: In this experiment, the test colour obtained by the reaction of heavy metal impurities with saturated solution of hydrogen sulphide is compared with standard colour obtained by the reaction of known quantity of lead with saturated solution of hydrogen sulphide.

$$Pb \quad + \quad H_2S \quad \longrightarrow \quad PbS \downarrow \quad + \quad 2\,H^+$$
$$\text{colour (brown)}$$

The precipitate of heavy metal sulphide formed gives colour. Dilute acetic acid and ammonia are used to maintain pH between 3.0 and 4.0 so that the precipitate formed is colloidal and uniform. The saturated solution of hydrogen sulphide has to be prepared freshly for the experiment. Here hydrogen sulphide gas is generated using a specially devised apparatus called as Kipp's apparatus in which ferrous sulphide sticks are made to react with equal volumes of concentrated hydrochloric acid and water. Indian pharmacopoeia 1996, provides four methods depending on the resulting solution of substance (i.e., based on solubility, colour etc). Method A uses hydrogen sulphide solution, method B uses hydrogen sulphide solution after igniting the substance, method C uses sodium sulphide solution after treating the substance with sodium hydroxide solution, and in method D thioacetamide solution is used. In a concise way, the methods can be categorized as follows:

Method I: It is used for the substance which gives a clear, colorless solution under specified conditions.

Method II: It is used for the substance which does not give a clear, colorless solution.

Method III: It is used for the substance which gives a clear, colorless solution in sodium hydroxide medium.

Procedure:

Test colour: Dissolve the given sample in 25 ml of water and transfer into a Nessler cylinder. Adjust with dilute acetic acid or dilute ammonia solution to a pH between 3.0 and 4.0, dilute with water to about 35 ml and mix. Add 10 ml of freshly prepared hydrogen sulphide solution, mix, dilute to 50 ml with water, allow to stand for 5 minutes and view downwards over a white surface.

Standard colour: Pipette 1.0 ml of lead standard solution (20 ppm Pb) into a Nessler cylinder and dilute with water to 25 ml. Adjust with dilute acetic acid or dilute ammonia solution to a pH between 3.0 and 4.0, dilute with water to about 35 ml and mix. Add 10 ml of freshly prepared hydrogen sulphide solution, mix, dilute to 50 ml with water, allow to stand for 5 minutes and view downwards over a white surface.

Method I: It is used for the substance which gives a clear, colorless solution under specified conditions.

Test solution	Standard solution
The sample solution is prepared as per the monograph and 25 ml of solution is transferred into a Nessler's cylinder.	Transfer 1.0 ml of standard lead solution and dilute to 25 ml with water.
Add dilute ammonia or acetic acid solution to adjust the pH between 3 to 4	Add dilute ammonia or acetic acid solution to adjust the pH between 3 to 4
Dilute to 35 ml with distilled water and mix well.	Dilute to 35 ml with distilled water and mix well.
Add 10 ml of freshly prepared hydrogen sulphide solution, mix, dilute to 50 ml with water.	Add 10 ml of freshly prepared hydrogen sulphide solution, mix, dilute to 50 ml with water.
Allow to stand for 5 min and view downwards over a white background.	Allow to stand for 5 min and view downwards over a white background.

Method II: It is used for the substance which does not give a clear, colorless solution.

Test solution	Standard solution
Transfer the prescribed quantity of sample into a crucible.	Transfer 1.0 ml of standard lead solution and dilute to 25 ml with water.
Moisten the sample with sulphuric acid and ignite on a low flame until complete charring of the sample.	Add dilute ammonia or acetic acid solution to adjust the pH between 3 to 4

Table Contd...

Test solution	Standard solution
Add 2 to 3 drops of nitric acid and heated to 500 °C and cool it.	Dilute to 35 ml with distilled water and mix well.
Then add 4 ml of dilute hydrochloric acid and digest for 2 min and evaporate to dryness. Then add 10 ml of dilute hydrochloric acid and digest the residue for two min.	Add 10ml of freshly prepared hydrogen sulphide solution, mix, dilute to 50 ml with water.
Neutralize with dilute ammonia solution and just acidified with acetic acid.	Allow to stand for 5 min and view downwards over a white background.
Adjust the pH 3 to 4, filter if necessary. Dilute to 35 ml with water.	
Add 10 ml of freshly prepared hydrogen sulphide solution. Dilute to 50 ml with water.	
Allow to stand for 5 min and view downwards over a white background.	

Method III: It is used for the substance which gives a clear, colorless solution in sodium hydroxide medium.

Test solution	Standard solution
The required quantity of sample is dissolved in 20 ml of water; add 5 ml of sodium hydroxide solution or the sample solution is prepared as per monograph.	The standard solution is prepared by using 1.0 ml of standard lead solution; add 5 ml of sodium hydroxide solution.
Make up to 50 ml with water.	Make up to 50 ml with water.
Add 5 drops of sodium sulphide solution mix well and kept aside for 5 min.	Add 5 drops of sodium sulphide solution mix well and kept aside for 5 min.
View downwards over a white background.	View downwards over a white background.

Observation:

If the color produced in the test solution is not more intense than that of standard solution, the sample complies with the standards of I.P or vice versa.

Test colour is not more intense than standard colour.

or

Test colour is more intense than standard colour.

Report/Result:

The given sample passes limit test for heavy metals.

or

The given sample fails limit test for heavy metals.

Preparation of Reagents:

1. *Dilute acetic acid:* Contains approximately 6% w/w of CH_3COOH. Dilute 57 ml of glacial acetic acid to 1000 ml with water.

2. *Dilute ammonia solution:* Contains approximately 10% w/w of NH_3. Dilute 425 ml of strong ammonia solution to 1000 ml. Store in well-closed containers in a cool place.

3. *Lead Standard solution (0.1% Pb):* Dissolve 0.400 g of lead nitrate in water containing 2 ml of nitric acid and add sufficient water to produce 250.0 ml.

4. *Lead Standard solution (100 ppm Pb):* Dilute 1 volume of lead standard solution (0.1% Pb) to 10 volumes with water.

5. *Lead Standard solution (20 ppm Pb):* Dilute 1 volume of lead standard solution (100 ppm Pb) to 5 volumes with water.

Experiment 05

Limit Test for Arsenic

Aim: To perform limit test for arsenic for the given sample.

Requirements: Arsenic apparatus, lead acetate cotton, mercuric chloride paper, 1 M potassium iodide solution, zinc dust (As T), water bath, arsenic standard solution (10 ppm As), 1 ml bulb pipette, 5 ml pipette, stannated hydrochloric acid.

Principle: In this experiment, the test stain obtained by the reaction of arsenic impurities in the form of arsine gas with mercuric chloride (paper) is compared with standard stain obtained by the reaction of known quantity of arsenic (in the form of arsine gas) with mercuric chloride.

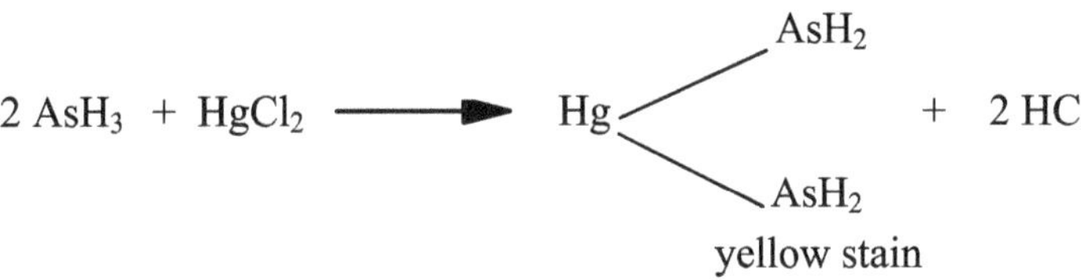

A specially designed apparatus is used for the limit test. In addition to the above product $AsH(HgBr)_2$, $As(HgBr)$ and As_2Hg_3 are formed which also form yellow or brown stain on the mercuric chloride paper.

Here, Arsenic present is converted to arsenic acid in acid. The arsenic acid is then reduced to arsenous acid.

$$H_3AsO_4 \longrightarrow H_3AsO_3$$
Arsenic acid   Arsenous acid

The nacent hydrogen produced by the reaction of zinc and hydrochloric acid reduces arsenous acid to arsine gas.

$$H_3AsO_3 + 3 H_2 \longrightarrow AsH_3\uparrow + 3 H_2O$$
Arsine gas

Lead acetate cotton is used to remove traces of hydrogen sulphide (in the arsine and hydrogen gas) which is formed due to presence of any sulphide impurities.

$$Pb(CH_3COO)_2 + H_2S \longrightarrow PbS \downarrow + 2\ CH_3COOH$$

The method is called the Gutzeit method (modified)

Stannated hydrochloric acid is used for steady and uniform liberation of hydrogen gas from zinc. Since, zinc is not very reactive toward hydrochloric acid, tin forms Sn/Zn couple and makes reaction of zinc and hydrochloric acid faster.

Stannous chloride present in stannated hydrochloric acid reduces arsenic (As^{5+}) to arsenous (As^{3+}). Hydrogen gas liberated also act as a carrier gas for arsine.

A side hole at the lower end of the tube in arsenic apparatus prevents condensed liquid from being forced up the tube by the pressure of hydrogen, thus preventing blockade. Potassium iodide is also added to reduce arsenic to arsenous.

Description of Apparatus:

The apparatus (see figure) consists of a 100 ml bottle or conical flask closed with a rubber or ground-glass stopper through which passes a glass tube (about 20 cm X 5 mm). The lower part of the tube is drawn to an internal diameter of 1.0 mm, and 15 mm from its tip is a lateral orifice 2 to 3 mm in diameter. When the tube is in position in the stopper the lateral orifice should be at least 3 mm below the lower surface of the stopper. The upper end of the tube has a perfectly flat surface at right angles to the axis of the tube. A second glass tube of the same internal diameter and 30 mm long, with a similar flat surface, is placed in contact with the first and is held in position by two spiral springs or clips. Into the lower tube insert 50 to 60 mg of lead acetate cotton, loosely packed, or a small plug of cotton and a rolled piece of lead acetate paper weighing 50 to 60 mg. Between the flat surfaces of the tubes place a disc or a small square of mercuric chloride paper large enough to cover the orifice of the tube (15 mm X 15 mm).

Diagram of Arsenic Apparatus:

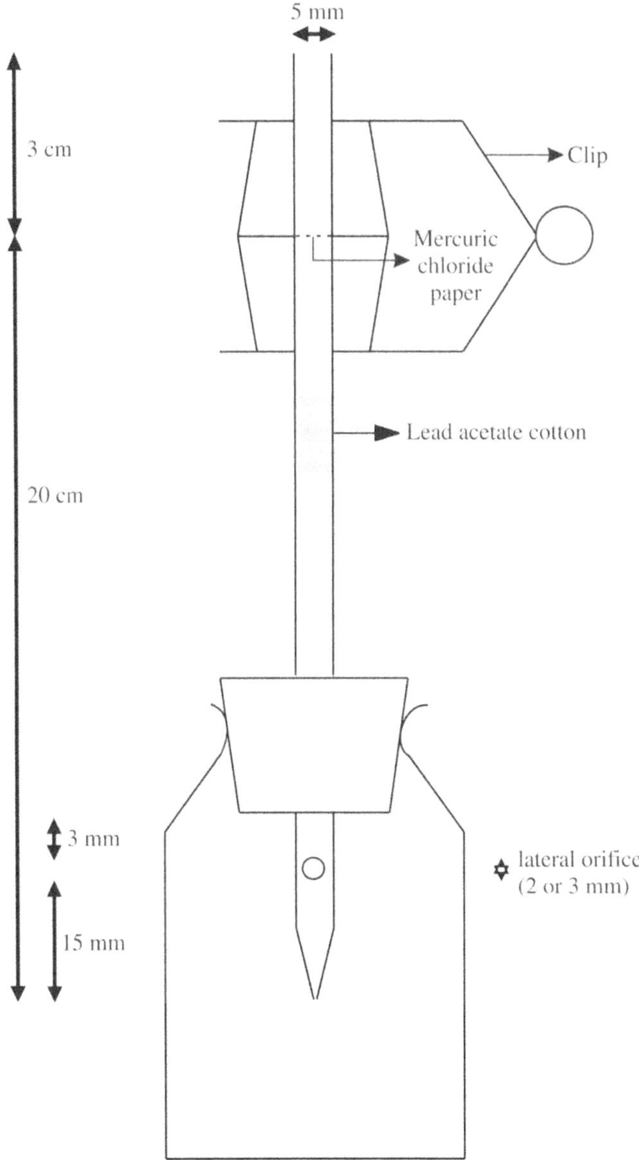

Procedure:

Test stain: Dissolve the given sample in 50 ml water and add 10 ml of stannated hydrochloric acid and transfer into the arsenic apparatus bottle. Add 5 ml of 1 M potassium iodide and 10 g of zinc AsT. Immediately assemble the apparatus and immerse the bottle in a water bath at a temperature such that a uniform evolution of gas is maintained. After 40 minutes observe the stain produced on the mercuric chloride paper.

Standard stain: Transfer 1.0 ml of arsenic standard solution into an arsenic apparatus bottle and dilute to 50 ml with water. Add 10 ml of stannated hydrochloric acid. Add 5 ml of 1 M potassium iodide and 10 g of zinc AsT. Immediately assemble the apparatus and immerse the bottle in a water bath at a temperature such that a uniform evolution of gas is maintained. After 40 minutes observe the stain produced on the mercuric chloride paper.

Observation:

Test stain is not more intense than standard stain.

or

Test stain is more intense than standard stain.

Report/Result:

The given sample passes limit test for arsenic.

or

The given sample fails limit test for arsenic.

Preparation of Reagents:

1. *1M potassium iodide:* Dissolve 166.0 g of potassium iodide in sufficient water to produce 1000 ml.

2. *2 M sodium hydroxide:* Solution of any molarity xM may be prepared by dissolving $40x$ of sodium hydroxide in sufficient water to produce 1000 ml.

3. *Arsenic standard solution (10 ppm As):* Dissolve 0.330 g of arsenic trioxide in 5 ml of 2 M sodium hydroxide and dilute to 250.0 ml with water. Dilute 1 volume of this solution to 100 volumes with water.

4. *Lead acetate cotton:* Immerse absorbent cotton in a mixture of 10 volumes of lead acetate solution and 1 volume of 2 M acetic acid. Drain off the excess of liquid by placing it on several layers of filter paper without squeezing the cotton. Allow to dry at room temperature. Store in tightly-closed containers.

5. *Lead acetate paper:* Prepare from lead acetate solution and dry the impregnated paper at 100°, avoiding contact with metal.

6. *Lead acetate solution:* A 10.0% w/v solution of lead acetate in carbon-di-oxide free water.

7. *Mercuric chloride paper:* Smooth white filter paper, not less than 25mm in width, soaked in a saturated solution of mercuric chloride, pressed to remove superfluous solution and dried at about 60° in the dark. The grade of filter paper is such that the weight is between 65 and 120 g per sq.m; the thickness in mm of 400 papers is approximately equal numerically, to the weight in g per sq.m.

8. *Stannated hydrochloric acid:* Stannated hydrochloric acid, low in arsenic, of commercial grade or prepared by adding 1 ml of stannous chloride solution AsT to 100 ml of hydrochloric acid AsT.

9. *Stannous chloride solution AsT:* Stannous chloride solution, low in arsenic, commercially available or prepared from stannous chloride solution by adding an equal volume of hydrochloric acid AsT, reducing to the original volume by boiling and filtering through a fine-grain filter paper.

Note: Use directly the sample in case of liquids.

Experiment 06

Limit Test for Lead

Aim: To perform limit test for lead for the given sample.

Requirements: Ammonium citrate solution Sp, hydroxyl amine hydrochloride solution Sp, phenol-red solution, strong ammonia solution, potassium cyanide solution Sp, dithizone extraction solution, 1% v/v solution of nitric acid, chloroform, dithizone standard solution, lead standard solution (1 ppm Pb), separating flasks, beakers, separating flask ring, test tubes.

Principle: In this experiment, the test colour in chloroform layer obtained by the reaction of lead impurities with diphenyl thiocarbazone (dithizone) is compared with standard colour in chloroform layer obtained by the reaction of known quantity of lead with diphenyl thiocarbazone (dithizone).

Dithizone in chloroform, extracts lead from alkaline aqueous solution as lead dithizone complex (violet in colour).

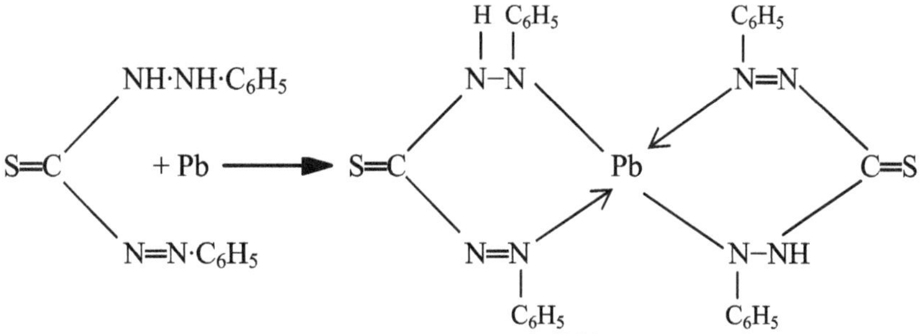

$$
\underset{\text{Lead dithionate complex}}{
\begin{array}{c}
\text{NH·NH·C}_6\text{H}_5 \\
S{=}C \\
\text{N}{=}\text{N·C}_6\text{H}_5
\end{array}
+ \text{Pb} \longrightarrow
\begin{array}{c}
\text{H} \quad \text{C}_6\text{H}_5 \\
\text{N--N} \\
S{=}C \qquad \text{Pb} \\
\text{N}{=}\text{N} \\
\text{C}_6\text{H}_5
\end{array}
\begin{array}{c}
\text{C}_6\text{H}_5 \\
\text{N}{=}\text{N} \\
\qquad \text{C}{=}\text{S} \\
\text{N--NH} \\
\text{C}_6\text{H}_5
\end{array}
}
$$

In this experiment, ammonium citrate, potassium cyanide, hydroxylamine hydrochloride are used to extract and discard any interfering metal ions (other than lead) at optimum pH in the form of complex.

The original dithizone has green colour in chloroform, thus lead-dithizone shows violet colour. Intensity of the colour depends upon the amount of lead in the solution. Here basically, the sample dissolved in water after adding the reagents as per the procedure are made to extract with dithizone extract solution. The dithizone extract solution is separated (in chloroform) from water layer and a fresh dithizone extract solution is added to the previously extracted sample solution and then re-extracted and then organic layer separated from aqueous layer. The organic layer i.e., di-thizone lead complex layer is combined with the first. The procedure of extraction is continued until freshly taken di-thizone extract solution on extraction with sample solution does not give any violet colour indicating that all the lead has been extracted from the sample. Now all the combined chloroform layers containing lead-thizone complex (violet) is extracted with an aqueous solution of nitric acid so that the lead is now extracted from chloroform layer into aqueous layer by forming lead nitrate (soluble in water). After extracting with nitric acid, the combined di-thizone extraction solutions can be discarded since the lead is no more in the organic layer. Now the aqueous solution is extracted with exactly 5 ml of dithizone standard solution, separated and compared with standard solution. One has to keep in mind that the volume of di-thizone extract solution for extraction need not be accurate but has to take exactly 5 ml of di-thizone standard solution for colour comparison.

Procedure:

Test colour: Dissolve the given sample (as specified in the monograph) in water and transfer into a separator, add 6 ml of ammonium citrate solution Sp. and 2 ml of hydroxylamine hydrochloride solution Sp. Add two drops of phenol red solution and make the solution just alkaline (red in colour) by the addition of strong ammonia solution. Cool the solution if necessary and add 2 ml of potassium cyanide solution Sp. Immediately extract the solution with several quantities, each of 5 ml of dithizone extraction solution, draining off each extract into another separating funnel, until the dithizone extraction solution retains its green colour. Shake the combined dithizone solutions for 30 seconds with 30 ml of a 1% v/v solution of nitric acid and discard the chloroform layer. Add to the acid solution exactly 5 ml of dithizone standard solution and shake for 30 seconds. Observe the colour of chloroform layer.

Standard colour: Transfer a volume of lead standard solution (1ppm Pb) equivalent to the amount of lead permitted in the substance being examined into a separator, add 6 ml of ammonium citrate solution Sp. and 2 ml of hydroxylamine hydrochloride solution Sp. Add two drops of phenol red solution and make the solution just alkaline (red in colour) by the addition of strong ammonia solution. Cool the solution if necessary and add 2 ml of potassium cyanide solution Sp. Immediately extract the solution with several quantities, each of 5 ml of dithizone extraction solution, draining off each extract into another separating funnel, until the dithizone extraction solution retains its green colour. Shake the combined dithizone solutions for 30 seconds with 30 ml of a 1% v/v solution of nitric acid and discard the chloroform layer. Add to the acid solution exactly 5 ml of dithizone standard solution and shake for 30 seconds. Observe the colour of chloroform layer.

Test solution	Standard solution
The required quantity of sample is dissolved in water and transferred into a separating funnel.	Transfer required amount of lead standard solution (1 ppm lead) equivalent to the amount of lead permitted in the substance being examined into a separating funnel
Add 6 ml of ammonium citrate solution (Sp).	Add 6 ml of ammonium citrate solution (Sp).
Add 2 ml of hydroxylamine hydrochloride solution (Sp), and add two drops of phenol red solution.	Add 2 ml of hydroxylamine hydrochloride solution (Sp), and add two drops of phenol red solution.
Make the solution just alkaline by the addition of strong ammonia solutions cool it if necessary.	Make the solution just alkaline by the addition of strong ammonia solution cool it if necessary.
Add 2 ml of potassium cyanide solution (Sp).	Add 2 ml of potassium cyanide solution (Sp).
Extract immediately with several quantities, each of 5 ml of dithizone extraction solution until it becomes green.	Extract immediately with several quantities, each of 5 ml of dithizone extraction solution until it becomes green.
Combine the dithizone extracts and shaken for 30 seconds with 30 ml of 1 % v/v solution of nitric acid and discard the chloroform layer. (Dithizone remains in chloroform layer, lead nitrate in aqueous layer).	Combine the dithizone extracts and shaken for 30 seconds with 30 ml of 1 % v/v solution of nitric acid and discard the chloroform layer (dithizone remains in chloroform layer, lead nitrate in aqueous layer).
To this acid solution add 5 ml of standard dithizone solution.	To this acid solution add 5 ml of standard dithizone solution.
Shake well for 30 min and observe the color of chloroform layer after separation.	Shake well for 30 min and observe the color of chloroform layer after separation.

Observation:

Test colour of the chloroform layer is not more intense than standard colour of the chloroform layer.

or

Test colour of the chloroform layer is more intense than standard colour of the chloroform layer.

Report/Result:

The given sample passes limit test for lead.

or

The given sample fails limit test for lead.

Preparation of Reagents:

1. *1% v/v nitric acid:* Dilute 1 vol of nitric acid to 100 volumes with water.

2. *Ammonium citrate solution Sp:* Dissolve 40 g of citric acid in 90 ml of water, add 2 drops of phenol red solution and then add slowly strong ammonia solution until the solution acquires a reddish colour. Remove any lead present by extracting the solution with successive quantities, each of 30 ml, of dithizone extraction solution until the dithizone solution retains its orange-green colour.

3. *Dithizone extraction solution:* Dissolve 30 mg of dithizone in 1000 ml of chloroform and add 5 ml of ethanol (95%). Store the solution in a refrigerator. Before use, shake a suitable volume of the solution with about half its volume of a 1%v/v solution of nitric acid and discard the acid.

4. *Dithizone standard solution:* Dissolve 10 mg of dithizone in 1000 ml of chloroform. Store the solution in a glass-stoppered, lead-free, light-resistant bottle in a refrigerator.

5. *Hydroxylamine hydrochloride solution Sp:* Dissolve 20 g of hydroxylamine hydrochloride in sufficient water to produce about 65 ml. Transfer to a separator, add 5 drops of thymol blue solution and strong ammonia solution until the solution becomes yellow. Add 10 ml of a 4 % w/v solution of sodium di-ethyl-di-thio carbamate and allow to stand for 5 minutes. Extract with successive quantities, each of 10 ml of chloroform until a 5 ml portion of the extract does not acquire a yellow colour when shaken with dilute cupric sulphate solution. Add dilute hydrochloric acid until the solution is pink and then with sufficient water to produce 100 ml.

6. *Lead standard solution (0.1% Pb):* Dissolve 0.400 g of lead nitrate in water containing 2 ml of nitric acid and add sufficient water to produce 250.0 ml.

7. *Lead standard solution (1 ppm Pb):* Dilute 1 volume of lead standard solution (10 ppm Pb) to 10 volumes with water.

8. *Lead standard solution (10 ppm Pb):* Dilute 1 volume of lead standard solution (100 ppm Pb) to 10 volumes with water.

9. *Lead standard solution (100 ppm Pb):* Dilute 1 volume of lead standard solution (0.1% Pb) to 10 volumes with water.

10. *Potassium cyanide solution Sp:* Dissolve 50 g of potassium cyanide in sufficient water to produce 100 ml. Remove the lead from this solution by extraction with successive quantities, each of 20 ml of dithizone extraction solution until the dithizone solution retains its orange green colour. Extract any dithizone remaining in the cyanide solution by shaking with chloroform. Dilute this cyanide solution with sufficient water to produce a solution containing 10 g of potassium cyanide in each 100 ml.

11. *Strong ammonia solution:* (ammonia solution, strong) Contains 25.0% w/w of NH_3 (limits, 24.5 to 25.5); wt. per ml about 0.91 g; strength about 13.5 M. Store in well-closed containers in a cool place.

Note: Use directly the sample in case of liquids.

Experiment 07

Limit Test for Chlorides for Water Insoluble Substances

Aim: To perform limit test for chlorides for water insoluble activated charcoal.

Requirements: Nessler cylinders, glass rod, measuring cylinders, 1ml bulb pipette, 10 ml bulb pipette, dilute nitric acid, 0.1 M silver nitrate, chloride standard solution (25 ppm Cl), test sample (activated charcoal).

Principle: In this experiment, the test opalescence obtained by the reaction of chloride impurities with silver nitrate is compared with standard opalescence obtained by the reaction of known quantity of chloride with silver nitrate. Dilute nitric acid is used to dissolve other impurities if present.

$$Cl^- \ + \quad AgNO_3 \quad \xrightarrow{\text{Dil . HNO}_3} \quad AgCl \downarrow \quad + \quad NO_3^-$$
$$\text{opalescence}$$

The precipitate silver chloride formed is insoluble in dilute nitric acid and gives opalescence.

Here, the main objective is to check for chloride impurity in charcoal and not as such charcoal. Usually chloride salts are soluble in water. When charcoal is treated with water, chloride salt gets dissolved, where as charcoal does not. Hence, the filterate of the suspension is used for limit test for chloride.

Procedure:

Test opalescence: Boil 3.0 g of the activated charcoal with 75 ml water for 5 minutes, cool. Dilute to 100.0 ml with water and filter. Transfer 6.0 ml of the filterate to a Nessler cylinder. Add 10 ml of dilute nitric acid, dilute to 50 ml with water. Add 1 ml of 0.1 M silver nitrate. Stir immediately with a glass rod and allow to stand for 5 minutes protected from light. View transversely against a black background.

Standard opalescence: Transfer 10.0 ml of chloride standard solution (25 ppm Cl) into a Nessler cylinder and add 5 ml of water. Add 10 ml of dilute nitric acid, dilute to 50 ml with water. Add 1 ml of 0.1 M silver nitrate. Stir immediately with a glass rod and allow to stand for 5 minutes protected from light. View transversely against a black background.

Observation:

Test opalescence is not more intense than standard opalescence.

or

Test opalescence is more intense than standard opalescence.

Report/Result:

The given sample passes limit test for chlorides.

or

The given sample fails limit test for chlorides.

Preparation of Reagents:

1. *0.1 M silver nitrate:* Dissolve 17.0 g of silver nitrate in sufficient water to 1000 ml. (Store in light-resistant containers)

2. *Chloride standard solution (25 ppm Cl):* Dilute 5 volumes of a 0.0824% w/v of sodium chloride to 100 volumes with water.

3. *Dilute nitric acid:* Contains approximately 10% w/w of HNO_3. Dilute 106 ml of nitric acid to 1000 ml with water.

Experiment 08

Limit Test for Chlorides for Coloured Substances

Aim: To perform limit test for chlorides for the given sample (potassium permanganate).

Requirements: Nessler cylinders, glass rod, measuring cylinders, 1ml bulb pipette, 10 ml bulb pipette, dilute nitric acid, 0.1 M silver nitrate, chloride standard solution (25 ppm Cl), test sample, ethanol (95%).

Principle: In this experiment, the test opalescence obtained by the reaction of chloride impurities with silver nitrate is compared with standard opalescence obtained by the reaction of known quantity of chloride with silver nitrate. Dilute nitric acid is used to dissolve other impurities if present.

$$Cl^- \ + \ AgNO_3 \ \xrightarrow{\ Dil . HNO_3\ } \ \underset{opalescence}{AgCl \downarrow} \ + \ NO_3^-$$

The precipitate silver chloride formed is insoluble in dilute nitric acid and gives opalescence.

Potassium permanganate in water possess purple colour. If limit test for chlorides is performed directly with potassium permanganate solution, the opalescence is not clearly observed due to colour of solution.   Hence, potassium permanganate having chloride impurities is made to react with ethanol during which acetic acid (oxidation of ethanol by potassium permanganate) and manganese dioxide (reduction of potassium permanganate) are produced. The resultant manganese dioxide suspension which on filteration, the filterate is colour less having the chloride impurity in it. This colour less filterate is used for the limit test for chloride.

$$KMnO_4 + CH_3CH_2OH \ \longrightarrow \ MnO_2 \downarrow + CH_3COOH \ + K^+$$

Procedure:

Test opalescence: Dissolve 1.5 g of the given sample in 50 ml of water, heat on a water-bath and add gradually 6 ml of ethanol (95%). Cool. Dilute to 60 ml with water and filter.   Transfer 40 ml of the filterate to a Nessler cylinder. Add 10 ml of dilute nitric acid. Add 1 ml of 0.1 M silver nitrate. Stir immediately with a glass rod and allow to stand for 5 minutes protected from light. View transversely against a black background.

Standard opalescence: Transfer 10.0 ml of chloride standard solution (25 ppm Cl) into a Nessler cylinder and add 5 ml of water. Add 10 ml of dilute nitric acid, dilute to 50 ml with water. Add 1 ml of 0.1 M silver nitrate. Stir immediately with a glass rod and allow to stand for 5 minutes protected from light. View transversely against a black background.

Test solution	Standard solution
Transfer 1.5gm of the sample into a 100ml beaker and add 50ml of distilled water. Heat it on a water bath.	Transfer 10.0 ml of standard chloride solution (25 ppm) in to a Nessler's cylinder and add 5 ml water.
To this, slowly add 6 ml of ethyl alcohol. Dilute to 60 ml with water. Cool the solution, filter and then collect the filtrate.	Add 10 ml of dilute nitric acid, dilute to 50 ml with water.
Transfer 40ml of filtrate into a Nessler's cylinder and add 10ml of dilute nitric acid. Add 1ml of 0.1M silver nitrate solution.	Add 1 ml of 0.1 M silver nitrate solution.
Stir immediately with a glass rod and allowed to stand for 5 min, protected from light and viewed transversely against a black background.	Stir immediately with a glass rod and allowed to stand for 5 min, protected from light and viewed transversely against a black background.

Observation:

Test opalescence is not more intense than standard opalescence.

or

Test opalescence is more intense than standard opalescence.

Report/Result:

The given sample passes limit test for chlorides.

or

The given sample fails limit test for chlorides.

Preparation of Reagents:

1. *0.1 M silver nitrate*: Dissolve 17.0 g of silver nitrate in sufficient water to 1000 ml. (Store in light-resistant containers)

2. *Chloride standard solution (25 ppm Cl)*: Dilute 5 volumes of a 0.0824% w/v of sodium chloride to 100 volumes with water.

3. *Dilute nitric acid:* Contains approximately 10% w/w of HNO_3.

   Dilute 106 ml of nitric acid to 1000 ml with water.

Experiment 09

Limit Test for Chlorides in Sodium Benzoate

Aim: To perform the limit test for chlorides for the given sample of sodium benzoate and report its compliance /non compliance with standards of I.P.

Requirements:

The given sample, 0.1M silver nitrate solution, dilute nitric acid, distilled water, standard chloride solution (25 ppm) and sodium carbonate solution (0.5 M), Nessler's cylinder, glass rod, bulb pipette (1ml and 10 ml), standard flask and measuring cylinders.

Principle: Sodium benzoate is insoluble in water. If any chloride impurities are present in the sample, they are soluble in water and gives the opalescence when treated with silver nitrate. This test is performed by heating the sample with sodium carbonate solution until charring occurs and dissolve the residue in dilute nitric acid and water. The resulting mixture is filtered and the filtrate obtained is used for performing the limit test.

Limit test for chloride is based upon the reaction of chloride impurities with silver nitrate in the presence of dilute nitric acid. The turbidity/opalescence produced in the test solution is compared with the standard turbidity/opalescence produced or obtained by the reaction of known quantity of chloride with silver nitrate.

$$Cl^- \;+\; AgNO_3 \xrightarrow{\text{Dilute } HNO_3} AgCl\downarrow \;+\; NO_3^-$$
$$\text{opalescence/Turbidity}$$

$$Na_2CO_3 + 2Cl^- + 2H^+ \longrightarrow 2NaCl + H_2O + CO_2$$

The silver chloride precipitate formed is insoluble in dilute nitric acid which gives turbidity/opalescence.

Reasons: 1.Dilute nitric acid is used to dissolve other impurities if present.

Procedure:

Test solution	Standard solution
Transfer 0.33 gm of sample in to a beaker. To this add 5 ml of 0.5 M sodium carbonate solution.	Transfer 10 ml of standard chloride solution (25 ppm) in to a Nessler's cylinder and add 5 ml water.

Table *Contd...*

Test solution	Standard solution
Evaporate to dry the mixture, heat the residue at below 400 °C until complete charring occurs. Extract the residue with 10 ml of water and 12 ml of dilute nitric acid. Filter the extract, collect the filtrate. Transfer the filtrate in to a Nessler's cylinder. Add 10 ml of dilute nitric acid, dilute to 50 ml with water.	Add 10 ml of dilute nitric acid, dilute to 50 ml with water.
Add 1 ml of 0.1 M silver nitrate solution.	Add 1 ml of 0.1 M silver nitrate solution.
Stir immediately with a glass rod and allowed to stand for 5 mins, protected from light and viewed transversely against a black background.	Stir immediately with a glass rod and allowed to stand for 5 mins, protected from light and viewed transversely against a black background.

Observation and Inference:

If the opalescence /turbidity produced in the test solution is less than that of the standard solution, the given sample complies with the standards of I.P. or vice versa.

Report: The given sample complies / not complies with the standards of I.P.

Preparation of Reagents:

1. **0.1 M AgNO$_3$ solution**

   Dissolve 17 gm of silver nitrate in sufficient amount of distilled water to produce 1000 ml and stored in light resistant container.

2. **Dilute Nitric acid (10% w/w of HNO$_3$)**

   Dissolve 106 ml of nitric acid in distilled water to produce 1000ml.

3. **Chloride standard solution (25 ppm chloride)**

   Dissolve 0.0824 gm of sodium chloride in 100ml of distilled water (stock solution). Dilute 3ml of the above stock solution to 100ml with distilled water.

4. **Preparation of 0.5 M Sodium carbonate solution**

   Dissolve 143.75 gm of sodium carbonate in 1000 ml of water.

Experiment 10

Limit Test for Chlorides in Sodium Bicarbonate

Aim: To perform the limit test for chlorides for the given sample of sodium bicarbonate and report its compliance /non compliance with standards of I.P.

Requirements:

Test sample, 0.1M silver nitrate solution, dilute nitric acid, nitric acid (conc.) distilled water and standard chloride solution (25 ppm), Nessler's cylinder, glass rod, bulb pipette (1ml and 10 ml), standard flask and measuring cylinders.

Principle:

Limit test for chlorides is based upon the reaction of chloride impurities with silver nitrate in the presence of dilute nitric acid. The turbidity/opalescence produced in the test solution is compared with the standard turbidity/ opalescence produced or obtained by the reaction of known quantity of chloride with silver nitrate.

$$Cl^- \;+\; AgNO_3 \;\xrightarrow{\text{Dilute } HNO_3}\; AgCl\downarrow \;+\; NO_3^-$$
$$\text{opalescence/Turbidity}$$

The silver chloride precipitate formed is insoluble in dilute nitric acid which gives turbidity/opalescence.

Reasons: 1.Dilute nitric acid is used to dissolve other impurities if present.

Procedure:

Test solution	Standard solution
Dissolve 1.25g of sample in 15 ml water and transfer in to Nessler's cylinder.	Transfer 10 ml of standard chloride solution (25 ppm) in to a Nessler's cylinder and add 5 ml water.
Then add 2 ml of nitric acid, dilute to 50 ml with water.	Add 10 ml of dilute nitric acid, dilute to 50 ml with water.
Add 1 ml of 0.1 M silver nitrate solution.	Add 1 ml of 0.1 M silver nitrate solution.
Stir immediately with a glass rod and allowed to stand for 5 mins, protected from light and viewed transversely against a black background.	Stir immediately with a glass rod and allowed to stand for 5 mins, protected from light and viewed transversely against a black background.

Observation and Inference:

If the opalescence /turbidity produced in the test solution is less than that of the standard solution, the given sample complies with the standards of I.P. or vice versa.

Report: The given sample complies / not complies with the standards of I.P.

Preparation of Reagents:

1. **0.1 M AgNO$_3$ solution**

   Dissolve 17gm of silver nitrate in sufficient amount of distilled water to produce 1000 ml and stored in light resistant container.

2. **Dilute Nitric acid (10% w/w of HNO$_3$)**

   Dissolve 106 ml of nitric acid in distilled water to produce 1000ml.

3. **Chloride standard solution (25 ppm chloride)**

   Dissolve 0.0824 gm of sodium chloride in 100ml of distilled water (stock solution). Dilute 5 ml of the above stock solution to 100 ml with distilled water.

2

Preparation of In-Organic Compounds

Introduction

Several in-organic compounds are used as drugs in human ailments. The critical problem with in-organic drug manufacturing is the solubility of desired and un-desired in-organic compounds in water. Atmost care has to be taken in the manufacture so that required product is obtained in required purity.

One has to have basic skills in handling preparation of various drugs at laboratory scale. As a basic point, for a better yield of a product, the reaction is necessarily to be carried out in homogenous solution.

The product obtained in the precipitate form, or on concentrating reaction mixture has to be thoroughly washed with cold water several times to wash away impurities minimizing less loss of desired product.

Several drugs like sodium nitroprusside, sodium nitrite, sodium thiosulphate are critical drugs used in emergency conditions. Several compounds like sodium chloride, potassium chloride, calcium chloride are used in electrolyte balance. A compound like sodium fluoride is used as dentrifice. Zinc chloride is used as pharmaceutical aid for insulin preparation. Zinc oxide, zinc sulphate are used as astringents. Zinc undecenoate is used as anti-fungal. Barium sulphate is used as diagnostic agent.

Experiment 11

Preparation of Boric Acid

Aim: To prepare and submit boric acid.

Requirements: Borax, sulphuric acid, beakers, spatula, porcelain plate, funnel, burner.

Principle: Boric acid is also called as ortho boric acid. It is a white crystalline powder or white crystals, odour less. According to IP 1996, it contains not less than 99.5% and not more than 100.5% of H_3BO_3, calculated with reference to dried substance.

Other than solubility and identification tests, IP 1996 specifies tests for pH, clarity and colour of solution, solubility in ethanol, arsenic, heavy metals, sulphates, loss on drying, assay.

Boric acid is estimated (assayed) quantitatively by titrating with 1M sodium hydroxide in presence of glycerine using phenolphthalein as indicator (acid-base titration).

Boric acid is prepared by treating hot solution of borax in water with either sulphuric acid or hydrochloric acid. Hydrochloric acid is preferred when boric acid prepared is used for medicinal purpose. This is so because hydrochloric acid is a gas when compared with sulphuric acid.

$$Na_2B_4O_7 + 2\ HCl + 5\ H_2O \rightarrow 2\ NaCl + 4\ H_3BO_3 \downarrow$$
$$201 \qquad 36.5 \quad 18 \qquad 58.44 \quad 61.83$$

$$Na_2B_4O_7 + H_2SO_4 + 5\ H_2O \rightarrow Na_2SO_4 + 4\ H_3BO_3 \downarrow$$
$$201 \qquad 98.07 \quad 18 \qquad 142.04 \quad 61.83$$

Here, 1 mole of borax reacts with 2 moles of hydrochloric acid or 1 mole of sulphuric acid.

The boric acid prepared must be thoroughly washed with water to remove chloride or sulphate impurities which are imparted from bi-products.

Procedure:

Dissolve the required quantity of borax in minimum water. Warm if necessary. To the homogenous solution add drop wise hydrochloric acid during which a white suspension is formed. The suspension is filtered and the crude boric acid on the filter paper is thoroughly washed until no chloride impurities in the washings. The crude boric acid is re-crystallized using hot water. The product obtained is dried and weighed.

Calculations:

Theoretical yield : 201 g of borax gives → 4 x 61.83 g of boric acid.

X g of borax gives → ? (say Y)

Theoretical yield (Y) = (X/201) × 4 × 61.83 = g

Practical yield =   g

Percentage yield (% yield) = (Practical yield/Theoretical yield) × 100 = %

Report: Percentage yield of boric acid =   %

Uses:

1. Local anti-infective, bacteriostatic.
2. Inactivate protein by precipitation, complexation.
3. 2.5-4.5% solutions are used as eye wash, mouth wash.
4. In treatment of diaper rash as an emollient antiseptic ointment.
5. Dusting powder.
6. Prevents discolouration of physostigmine solutions.
7. Solutions are used in irrigating of organs.
8. Buffer in epinephrine bitartarate ophthalmic solutions.

Storage: Store in a well closed container.

Experiment 12

Preparation of Sodium Citrate

Aim: To prepare and submit sodium citrate.

Requirements: Citric acid, sodium bicarbonate or sodium carbonate, beakers, spatula, porcelain plate, funnel, burner.

Principle: Sodium citrate is also called as tri-sodium citrate, tri-sodium 2-hydroxy propane-1, 2, 3-tricarboxylate dehydrate. It is white, granular crystals or white, crystalline powder, odourless, slightly deliquescent in moist air. According to IP 1996, it contains not less than 99.0% and not more than 101.0% of $C_6H_5Na_3O_7$, calculated with reference to the anhydrous substance.

Other than solubility and identification tests, IP 1996 specifies tests for acidity or alkalinity, clarity and colour of solution, arsenic, heavy metals, chlorides, oxalate, sulphate, tartarate, readily carbonisable substances, water and assay.

Sodium citrate is estimated (assayed) quantitatively by titrating with 0.1 M perchloric acid using 1-naphthol benzein solution as indicator (non-aqueous titration).

Sodium citrate is prepared by neutralizing a solution of citric acid with sodium carbonate or sodium bicarbonate.

$$
\begin{array}{c}
CH_2COOH \\
| \\
HO-C-COOH \\
| \\
CH_2COOH \\
192
\end{array}
\ + \ 3NaHCO_3 \ + \ 2H_2O
\ \longrightarrow \
\begin{array}{c}
CH_2COONa \\
| \\
HO-C-COONa \\
| \\
CH_2COONa \\
214
\end{array}
\ 2H_2O \ + \ 3CO_2 \ + \ 3H_2O
$$

with $3NaHCO_3$ (84) and $2H_2O$ (18).

$$
2\begin{array}{c}
CH_2COOH \\
| \\
HO-C-COOH \\
| \\
CH_2COOH \\
192
\end{array}
\ + \ 3NaHCO_3 \ + \ 2H_2O
\ \longrightarrow \
2\begin{array}{c}
CH_2COONa \\
| \\
HO-C-COONa \\
| \\
CH_2COONa \\
214
\end{array}
\ 2H_2O \ + \ 3CO_2 \ + \ 3H_2O
$$

with $3NaHCO_3$ (106) and $2H_2O$ (18).

Procedure:

Dissolve the required quantity of citric acid in water and add a aqueous solution of sodium bicarbonate to the citric acid solution during which carbon-dioxide gas is evolved as effervescence. After complete addition of sodium bicarbonate solution, ensure the solution is neutral and concentrate the solution with minimum solvent left behind. Cool and the crystals obtained are filtered, recrystallized with water, dried and submitted.

Calculations:

Theoretical yield : 192 g of citric acid gives $\rightarrow$ 214 g of sodium citrate.

$$X \text{ g of citric acid gives} \rightarrow ? \text{ (say Y)}$$

Theoretical yield (Y) = (X/192) $\times$ 214 =   g

Practical yield =   g

Percentage yield (% yield) = (Practical yield/Theoretical yield) $\times$ 100 =   %

Report: Percentage yield of sodium citrate =   %

Uses:

1.   Systemic antacid (1-4 g).
2.   Anti-coagulant by chelation of serum calcium.
3.   In expectorant preparation (1-2 g).
4.   As systemic alkalizer, urinary alkalizer.
5.   Solution (3%) is used to wash out syringes and apparatus before collection of blood.
6.   Mobilize calcium from the bone, and increase its renal excretion.
7.   Diuretic effect due to increased salt concentration.
8.   In chronic acidosis, administration of sodium citrate causes formation of CO_2 and bicarbonate (through Kreb's cycle), thus restore bicarbonate reserve.

Dose: 1 to 10 g

Storage: Stored in tightly closed containers.

Experiment 13

Preparation of Potash Alum

Aim: To prepare and submit potash alum.

Requirements: Potassium sulphate, aluminium sulphate, beakers, funnel, porcelain plate, spatula.

Principle: Potash alum is a sulphate salt of potassium and aluminium in the hydrated form. In general, alum has general formula $X_2SO_4.Y_2(SO_4)_3.24H_2O$ or $X^+.Y^{3+}.(SO_4^-)_2.12H_2O$, where x and y represent mono and trivalent metal cations respectively. Nine possible alums can be prepared. The best known are

Potash alum- $K_2SO_4.Al_2(SO_4)_3.24H_2O$

Ammonium alum- $AlNH_4(SO_4)_2.12H_2O$

Iron alum-$(NH_4)_2SO_4.Fe(SO_4)_3.24H_2O$

Chrome alum-$K_2SO_4.Cr_2(SO_4^-)_3.24H_2O$

Potash alum is used as astringent i.e., as protein precipitant in minor cuts to stop bleeding immediately.

According to IP 1965, Alum (potash alum) contains not less than 99.5% of $KAl(SO_4)_2.12H_2O$. Alum is a white powder or transparent, granular crystals, odourless with sweetish astringent taste. When heated, it melts and at about 200 ºC loses its water of crystallization with the formation of the anhydrous salt.

All types of alum form octahedral form of crystals and hence alums are isomorphous.

Other than solubility and identification tests, IP 1965 specifies tests for arsenic, heavy metals, iron, zinc and ammonia salts.

Alum is estimated gravimetrically by precipitating with ammonium chloride and ammonia into the form of Al_2O_3 (gravimetric).

Potash alum is prepared by mixing solutions of potassium sulphate and aluminium sulphate in water.

$$K_2SO_4 + Al_2(SO_4)_3 + 24\ H_2O \rightarrow K_2SO_4.Al_2(SO_4)_3.24H_2O \text{ or}$$

$$2\ KAl(SO_4)_2.12H_2O$$

174.25   342.38   18   948.44   474.4

Here 1 mole of aluminium sulphate and 1 mole of potassium sulphate gives 2 moles of alum.

Procedure:

Dissolve separately required quantity of potassium sulphate and aluminium sulphate in minimum water. Warm the solutions if necessary. The homogenous solutions are mixed and the resulting solution is left un-disturbed over night during which clear transparent crystals obtained were washed, recrystallised, dried and submitted.

Calculations:

Theoretical yield :

$$342 \text{ g of } Al_2(SO_4)_3 \text{ gives} \rightarrow 2 \times 474 \text{ g of } KAl(SO_4)_2.12H_2O.$$

$$X \text{ g of } Al_2(SO_4)_3 \text{ gives} \rightarrow ? \text{ (say Y)}$$

Theoretical yield (Y) = $(X/342) \times 2 \times 474 =$ g

Practical yield =   g

Percentage yield (% yield) = (Practical yield/Theoretical yield) $\times$ 100 =   %

Report: Percentage yield of potash alum =   %

Uses:

1. Astringent i.e. precipitate proteins.
2. In the preparation of toxoids, precipitated diphtheria.
3. Antiseptic.
4. Irrigation of urethra in the treatment of leucorrhoea.
5. Local styptic (stop bleeding).
6. Solutions (1-4%) used as mouth wash or gargle in stomatitis, pharyngitis.

Storage: Store in a tightly closed container.

Experiment 14

Preparation of Yellow Mercuric Oxide

Aim: To prepare and submit yellow mercuric oxide.

Requirements: Mercuric chloride, sodium hydroxide, beakers, funnel, porcelain plate, spatula.

Principle: Yellow mercuric oxide is also called as yellow precipitate. It is a orange-yellow, heavy, amorphous powder, odourless, stable in air but becomes discoloured on exposure to light.

According to IP 1965, it contains not less than 99.5% of HgO calculated with reference to the substance dried at 105°C for one hour.

Other than solubility and identification test, IP 1965 specifies tests for mercurous salts, chloride, loss on drying and sulphated residue.

Yellow mercuric oxide is estimated (assayed) by precipitate titration method using 0.1N ammonium thiocyanate using ferric ammonium sulphate as indicator.

It is prepared by treating concentrated solution of mercuric chloride in dilute solution of sodium hydroxide.

$$HgCl_2 + 2\,NaOH \rightarrow Hg(OH)_2 + 2\,NaCl$$
$$271.5 \qquad 40$$

$$Hg(OH)_2 \rightarrow \ HgO \downarrow + H_2O$$
$$216.59$$
$$\text{yellow}$$

Here 1 mole of mercuric chloride is reacting with 2 moles of sodium hydroxide giving 1 mole of yellow mercuric oxide.

Procedure: Dissolve 0.3 g of NaOH in about 10 ml of water. Add solution of $HgCl_2$ in about 10 ml of water drop wise with stirring. The suspension obtained is allowed to settle down. The supernatant is decanted and filtered. The precipitate is thoroughly washed with water, dried, weighed and submitted.

Calculations:

Theoretical yield :

217.5 g of mercuric chloride gives $\rightarrow$ 216.59 g of yellow HgO

X g of mercuric chloride gives $\rightarrow$? (say Y)

Theoretical yield (Y) = (X/271.5) × 216.59 =   g

Practical yield =   g

Percentage yield (% yield) = (Practical yield/Theoretical yield) × 100 =   %

Report: Percentage yield of yellow mercuric oxide =   %

Uses:

1. Germicidal, diuretic, anti-fungal, disinfectant, anti-syphilitic.

2. Eye ointment is used in ophthalmology.

3. Ointment (1%) is used in mild inflammatory conditions to treat blepharitis and conjunctivitis.

4. Ointment (2%) used in eczema and other skin infections.

5. Pruritus.

6. Epidermatophytosis.

Storage: Store in well closed container, protected from light.

Experiment 15

Preparation of Ammoniated Mercury

Aim: To prepare and submit ammoniated mercury.

Requirements: Mercuric chloride, ammonia, beakers, funnel, porcelain plate, spatula.

Principle: Ammoniated mercury is also called as amino chloride of mercury because one amino group has replaced as atom chlorine from mercuric chloride. It is a white heavy amorphous powder, odour less, stable in air, darkens on exposure to light. It contains not less than 98.0% of NH_2HgCl.

Other than solubility and identifications tests, IP 1965 specifies tests for mercurous chloride, carbonates and sulphated ash.

It is estimated (assayed) by treating with potassium iodide, during which liberated alkalies, ammonia and potassium hydroxide are titrated with 0.1 N HCl using methyl orange as an indicator (acid-base titration).

Ammoniated mercury is prepared by treating solution of mercuric chloride with dilute ammonia solution.

$$HgCl_2 \; + \; NH_3 \longrightarrow Hg\begin{matrix} \diagup NH_2 \\ \diagdown Cl \end{matrix} \; + \; NH_4Cl$$

271.5   252.1

During the preparation, the precipitate ammoniated mercury formed should not be washed thoroughly, which may remove ammonium chloride and cause yellow colour to the product.

Here 1 mole of mercuric chloride reacts with 1 mole of ammonia and gives 1 mole of ammoniated mercury.

Procedure:

Dissolve the required quantity of mercuric chloride in water. Warm if necessary. To the homogenous solution add dropwise ammonia solution. The resulting precipitate is filtered and minimal washed with precaution so as to not to retain yellow colour to the product. The resulting product is dried, weighed and submitted.

Calculations:

Theoretical yield :

217.5 g of mercuric chloride gives→252.1 g of ammoniated mercury.

X g of mercuric chloride gives → ? (say Y)

Theoretical yield (Y) = (X/271.5) × 252.1 =   g

Practical yield =   g

Percentage yield (% yield) = (Practical yield/Theoretical yield) × 100 =   %

Report: Percentage yield of ammoniated mercury =   %

Uses:

1. Anti-infective agent in treatment of impetigo (an infectious skin disease).
2. In Staphylococcal skin infection.
3. In dermatomycoses.
4. In psoriasis.
5. In crab infestations.

Storage: Preserve in well closed container, protected from light.

Experiment 16

Preparation of Ferrous Sulphate

Aim: To prepare and submit ferrous sulphate.

Requirements: Iron filings, sulphuric acid, beakers, funnel, burner, spatula.

Principle: Ferrous sulphate is also called as green vitriol. It is bluish green crystals, crystalline powder, odourless, efflorescent in air. On exposure to moist air, the crystals rapidly oxidize and become brown. It contains not less than 98.0 % and not more than 105.0 % of $FeSO_4.7H_2O$.

Other than solubility and identification tests, IP 1996 specifies tests for pH, clarity of solution, arsenic, copper, lead, zinc, manganese and chloride.

It is estimated (assayed) by titrating with 0.1M ceric ammonium nitrate using 0.1 ml of ferroin solution as indicator (redox titration).

Ferrous sulphate is prepared by treating iron filings or powder with dilute/concentrated sulphuric acid.

$$Fe + H_2SO_4 \longrightarrow FeSO_4 + 1/2\ H_2 \uparrow$$
$$55.84 \quad\quad 98.07 \quad\quad\quad\quad 278.01$$

Here 1 mole of iron filing reacts with 1 mole of sulphuric acid giving 1 mole of ferrous sulphate.

Procedure:

To about 50-100 ml of water in a beaker add required amount of concentrated sulphuric acid. To the dilute acid solution, add in several small increments iron filings or powder during which vigorous effervescence of liberated hydrogen gas is observed. After complete addition of iron filings, the resulting suspension is left aside until complete cessation of effervescence or immediately filtered to separate un-reacted iron. The resulting filterate is concentrated until about 10 ml solvent is left behind and to this about 2-3 ml concentrated sulphuric acid is added so as to convert ferric (if any present) to ferrous. The filterate is further concentrated to half volume and cooled during which pale green crystalline substance obtained is filtered, washed with cold water, recrystallised with water, dried and submitted.

Calculations:

Theoretical yield :

55.84g of iron gives $\rightarrow$ 278.01g of ferrous sulphate.

X g of iron gives $\rightarrow$? (say Y)

Theoretical yield (Y) = (X/55.84) $\times$ 278.01 =   g

Practical yield =   g

Percentage yield (% yield) = (Practical yield/Theoretical yield) $\times$ 100 =   %

Report: Percentage yield of ferrous sulphate =   %

Uses:

1. Haematinic
2. Iron deficiency anaemia.

Experiment 17

Preparation of Copper Sulphate

Aim: To prepare and submit copper sulphate.

Requirements: Copper filings, sulphuric acid, beakers, funnel, burner, spatula.

Principle: Copper sulphate is also called as blue vitriol. It is blue triclinic prisms or blue, crystalline powder. It contains not less than 98.5 % and not more than the equivalent of 101.0 % of $CuSO_4.5H_2O$.

Other than solubility and identification tests, IP 1965 specifies tests for acidity and clarity of solution, arsenic, iron, lead and zinc.

It is estimated (assayed) by treating with potassium iodide, acetic acid and titrating with 0.1N sodium thiosulphate using starch solution as indicator (redox titration).

Copper sulphate is prepared by treating copper filings or powder with dilute/concentrated sulphuric acid.

$$Cu + H_2SO_4 \longrightarrow CuSO_4 + 1/2\ H_2 \uparrow$$
$$63.54 \quad 98.07 \qquad\qquad 249.7$$

Here 1 mole of copper filing reacts with 1 mole of sulphuric acid giving 1 mole of copper sulphate.

Procedure:

To about 50-100 ml of water in a beaker add required amount of concentrated sulphuric acid. To the dilute acid solution, add in several small increments copper filings or powder during which vigorous effervescence of liberated hydrogen gas is observed. After complete addition of copper filings, the resulting suspension is left aside until complete cessation of effervescence or immediately filtered to separate un-reacted copper. The filtrate is concentrated by evaporation of solvent until about 5-10 ml of volume and cooled during which blue crystalline substance obtained is filtered, washed with cold water, recrystallised with water, dried and submitted.

Calculations:

Theoretical yield: 63.54g of copper gives→249.7g of copper sulphate.

X g of copper gives → ? (say Y)

Theoretical yield (Y) = (X/63.54) × 249.7 =   g

Practical yield =   g

Percentage yield (% yield) = (Practical yield/Theoretical yield) × 100 =   %

Report: Percentage yield of copper sulphate =   %

Uses:

1. Astringent.
2. Anti-microbial.

Experiment 18

Preparation of Potassium Citrate

Aim: To prepare and report the percentage yield of Potassium citrate from citric acid.

Requirements:

Beakers, glass rod, funnel, china dish, burner, filter paper, Citric acid, Potassium bicarbonate/ Potassium carbonate, water.

Principle: It is otherwise called as tri- Potassium citrate or tri potassium-2-hydroxy propane 1,2,3-tricarboxylate dehydrate. It is prepared by neutralization reaction between citric acid and potassium bicarbonate/ potassium carbonate.

Here citric acid reacts with potassium bicarbonate/ potassium carbonate to give potassiumcitrate.

$$3\,KHCO_3 + \underset{\substack{\text{Citric acid}\\192}}{HO-\overset{\displaystyle CH_2COOH}{\underset{\displaystyle CH_2COOH}{C}}-COOH} \longrightarrow \underset{324.4}{HO-\overset{\displaystyle CH_2COOK}{\underset{\displaystyle CH_2COOK}{C}}-COOH.\,H_2O} + 3\,CO_2\uparrow + 3\,H_2O$$

Potassium bicarbonate
100.12

$$3\,K_2CO_3 + \underset{\substack{\text{Citric acid}\\192}}{HO-\overset{\displaystyle CH_2COOH}{\underset{\displaystyle CH_2COOH}{C}}-COOH} \longrightarrow \underset{324.4}{HO-\overset{\displaystyle CH_2COOK}{\underset{\displaystyle CH_2COOK}{C}}-COOK.\,H_2O} + 3\,CO_2\uparrow + 3\,H_2O$$

Potassium bicarbonate
138.21

Procedure:

1. Dissolve 1.921 gm of citric acid and 4.15 gm of potassium bicarbonate in water separately.
2. Heat both the solutions.
3. The hot solution of citric acid is gradually added to the solution of potassium bicarbonate/ potassium carbonate solution until effervescence ceases(CO_2 gas is evolved).
4. After completion of addition, the pH of the solution should be maintained neutral.
5. Concentrate the solution with minimum quantity solvent left behind.

6. Cool, the crystals of potassium citrate obtained are filtered, dried and weighed. The crystals obtained should be neutral to phenolphthalein.

7. Recrystallisaton: The crystals obtained are recrystallised with hot water.

Calculations: Calculation of Theoretical Yield

192.1 gm of citric acid yields ----- > 324 gm of potassium citrate monohydrate.

1.921 gm of citric acid yields ----- > X gm.

$$X = \frac{1.921 \times 324}{192.1} = 3.24 \text{ gm}$$

Theoretical yield = 3.24 g.

Practical yield = ------------- gm.

$$\text{Percentage yield} = \frac{\text{Practical yield}}{\text{Theoretical yield}} \times 100$$

$$= \frac{\text{gm}}{3.24} \times 100$$

$$= \text{-------}\%$$

Report: The crystallized product of potassium citrate is prepared and submitted.

Practical yield	=	gm
Theoretical yield	=	gm
Percentage yield	=	%

Uses:

1. It is mainly used for its osmotic diuretic and diaphoretic action which is greater than other alkaline salts and ammonium compound.

2. It is also used as a systemic alkalising agent and having slight laxative action.

3. It is used as an anticoagulant.

Dose: 4 to 10 gm.

Storage: It should be stored in well closed containers, protected from moisture.

Note: When water of crystallization is taken into consideration, consider as potassium citrate monohydrate. It's molecular weight is 324.

Experiment 19

Preparation of Magnesium Sulphate

Aim: To prepare and submit the percentage yield of magnesium sulphate from magnesium carbonate or magnesium oxide or magnesium ribbon.

Requirements:

Beakers, funnels, glass rod, magnesium carbonate or magnesium oxide or magnesium ribbons and dilute sulphuric acid.

Principle: Magnesium sulphate is otherwise called as epsom salt. It is prepared by the neutralization reaction between magnesium carbonate or magnesium oxide or magnesium ribbon with dilute sulphuric acid. Here 1 mole of magnesium carbonate reacts with 1 mole of sulphuric acid and forms 1 mole of magnesium sulphate.

$$MgCO_3 \ + \ H_2SO_4 \ \longrightarrow \ MgSO_4 \ + \ H_2O \ + \ CO_2 \uparrow$$
$$84 \hspace{6cm} 120$$

$$Mg \ + \ H_2SO_4 \ \longrightarrow \ MgSO_4 \ + \ 1/2 \ H_2 \uparrow$$

$$MgO \ + \ H_2SO_4 \ \longrightarrow \ MgSO_4 \ + \ H_2O$$

Procedure:

1. Required quantity of magnesium carbonate (8 gm) / oxide/ magnesium ribbon is suspended in water.

2. To this add required quantity of hot, dilute sulphuric acid drop wise until effervescence ceases.

3. Filtered the solution and remove the unreacted materials, evaporate the filtrate until to dryness and collect the crystals.

Calculations:

Calculation of Theoretical Yield:

84 gm of magnesium carbonate $\rightarrow$ 120 gm of magnesium sulphate.

8 gm of magnesium carbonate $\rightarrow$ X gm

$$X = \frac{8 \times 120}{84} = 11.42 \text{ g}$$

Theoretical yield x = 11.42 gm

Practical yield = _______ gm.

$$\text{Percentage yield} = \frac{\text{Practical yield}}{\text{Theoretical yield}} \times 100$$

$$= \frac{\text{gm}}{11.42} \times 100$$

$$= \text{-----}\%$$

Report: The magnesium sulphate crystals are prepared and submitted.

Theoretical yield = ____ gm.

Practical yield = _____ gm.

Percentage yield = _____ %.

Uses:

1. The solution of magnesium sulphate is given by oral route which is used as an osmotic laxative and electrolyte replenishers.

2. It is given along with fruit juices due to its bitter taste and unpleasant odour.

3. It also used in renal function impaired patients as laxative.

Storage: It should be stored in tightly closed container and protected from moisture.

Experiment 20

Preparation of Aluminium Hydroxide

Aim: To prepare and submit aluminium hydroxide from aluminium sulphate and report its percentage yield.

Requirements:

Beakers, funnels, glass rod, aluminium sulphate, potash alum and sodium carbonate.

Principle: Aluminium hydroxide is prepared by the reaction between the hot solutions of potash alum with hot solution of sodium carbonate. During this reaction, potash alum reacts with sodium carbonate to give aluminium hydroxide, sodium sulphate, potassium sulphate and carbon dioxide gas is liberated.

$$3\,Na_2CO_3 + 2\,KAl(SO_4)_2\,12H_2O + 3\,H_2O \longrightarrow 2\,Al(OH)_3 \downarrow + 3\,Na_2SO_4 + K_2SO_4 + 3\,CO_2 \uparrow + 24\,H_2O$$
$$\;106 \qquad\quad 948.44 \qquad\qquad\qquad\qquad\qquad 78$$

Procedure:

1. Required quantity of potash alum (10 g) is dissolved in minimum amount of water and boil the solution.
2. Sodium carbonate solution is prepared by dissolving the required quantity of sample in minimum amount of water and boil the solution.
3. The hot solution of potash alum is added to the hot solution of sodium carbonate with constant stirring until the complete evolution of carbon dioxide gas, the aluminium hydroxide obtained settles down.
4. Filter the mixture, wash the precipitate by hot water, and dried it.

Calculations:

Calculation of theoretical yield:

948.44 gm of potash alum yields ---------- > 78 gm aluminium hydroxide.

10 gm of potash alum yields ------------- > X gm.

$$X = \frac{10}{948.44} \times 78 = 0.822 \text{ g}$$

Theoretical yield = 0.822 g.

Practical yield = -------------gm.

$$\text{Percentage yield} = \frac{\text{Practical yield}}{\text{Theoretical yield}} \times 100$$

$$= \frac{\text{gm}}{0.822} \times 100$$

$$= \text{--------}\%$$

Report: The aluminium hydroxide is prepared and submitted.

Practical yield	=	gm
Theoretical yield	=	gm
Percentage yield	=	%

Uses:

1. Aluminium hydroxide gel is very effective low acting antacid.

2. It has the advantage that it is not absorbed in the gastro intestinal tract (GIT) and doses not generate carbon dioxide and metallic carbonates.

3. It is used to absorb gastric toxins and gases.

Storage: It should be stored in well closed blue or amber colored container temperature of not exceeding to 30 $^{\circ}$C. Do not freeze it.

Experiment 21

Preparation of Barium Sulphate

Aim: To prepare and report the percentage yield of barium sulphate from barium chloride.

Requirements:

Barium chloride, sodium sulphate, beakers, funnels and glass rod

Principle: Barium sulphate is prepared by the precipitation reaction between the saturated solution of barium chloride and any soluble sulphates such as sodium sulphate. Barium sulphate is insoluble in water. Here 1 mole of barium chloride reacts with 1 mole of sodium sulphate to give 1 mole of barium sulphate.

$$BaCl \;+\; Na_2SO_4 \longrightarrow BaSO_4 \downarrow \;+\; 2\,NaCl$$

$$208.23 \qquad 142 \qquad\qquad 233$$

Procedure:

1. Dissolve the required quantity (2.083 gm) of barium chloride in minimum amount of water.

2. To the above solution add required quantity (1.4206gm) of sodium sulphate solution with continuous stirring.

3. Keep it stand for 5-10 minutes. The precipitate obtained is insoluble in water which is collected, washed with water and dried in a oven.

Calculations:

Calculation of theoretical yield:

208.3 gm of barium chloride yields ---------- > 233.4 gm of barium sulphate.

2.083 gm of barium chloride yields ------------- > X gm.

$$X = \frac{2.083 \times 233.4}{208.3} = 2.334 \text{ g}$$

Theoretical yield = 2.334 gm.

Practical yield = -------------gm.

$$\text{Percentage yield} = \frac{\text{Pr actical yield}}{\text{Theoretical yield}} \times 100$$

$$= \frac{\text{gm}}{2.334} \times 100$$

$$= \text{--------}\%$$

Report: The product barium sulphate is prepared and submitted.

Practical yield	=	gm
Theoretical yield	=	gm
Percentage yield	=	%

Uses:

1. Barium sulphate is used as a diagnostic agent (radio opaque contrast medium).

2. It is also used as a radio opaque contrast medium for x-ray determination of gastro intestinal tract (roentgenographic studies).

Note: Wash the Barium sulphate precipitate with water until the washings gives no precipitate with silver nitrate solution. This is to ensure that the end product is free from chloride impurities.

Experiment 22

Preparation of Zinc Oxide

Aim: To prepare and report the percentage yield of zinc oxide.

Requirements:

Zinc sulphate, sodium carbonate, beakers, crucible/china dish and glass rod.

Principle: Pure zinc oxide is obtained by the reaction between zinc sulphate and sodium carbonate solution to give zinc carbonate. The basic zinc carbonate obtained is ignited gently whereby it loses carbon dioxide to yields zinc oxide.

$$ZnSO_4.7H_2O \ \text{ or } \ ZnSO_4 \ + \ Na_2CO_3 \longrightarrow ZnCO_3 \ + \ Na_2SO_4$$

$$\quad 287.5 \qquad\qquad 161.47 \qquad 106 \qquad\qquad\qquad 125.42 \qquad 142$$

$$ZnCO_3 \ \xrightarrow{\ \Delta\ } \ ZnO \ + \ CO_2\uparrow$$

$$125 \qquad\qquad 81$$

Procedure:

1. Weight accurately about the required quantity of zinc sulphate (hepta hydrate) (2.875 gm) and dissolve it in minimum quantity of water.

2. Sodium carbonate solution is prepared by dissolving required amount of sample (1.06 gm) in minimum amount of water and boiling the solution.

3. The solution of zinc sulphate is gradually added to the boiling solution of sodium carbonate with constant stirring and keep it aside for 5-10 minutes.

4. The precipitated zinc carbonate is separated by filtration, washed with water until it free from sulphate impurities (Filtrate does not show the test for sulphate) and dried.

5. The precipitated zinc carbonate is slightly ignited until the complete evaluation of carbon dioxide gas to yield zinc oxide.

Calculations:

Calculation of theoretical yield:

287.5 gm of zinc sulphate yields ---------- > 81.4 of zinc oxide.

2.875 gm of zinc sulphate yields ------------- > X gm.

$$X = \frac{2.875 \times 81.4}{287.5} = 0.814 \text{ g}$$

Theoretical yield = 0.814 gm.

Practical yield = -------------gm.

$$\text{Percentage yield} = \frac{\text{Practical yield}}{\text{Theoretical yield}} \times 100$$

$$= \frac{\text{gm}}{0.814} \times 100$$

$$= \text{--------}\%$$

Report:

Practical yield	=	gm
Theoretical yield	=	gm
Percentage yield	=	%

Uses:

1. It mainly acts as mild astringent and topical protectant.
2. It is also used for the treatment of eczema, varicose, ulcers, psoriasis and various types of skin diseases.
3. In dentistry it is used as dental cement for temporary filling of teeth.
4. It is also used in the manufacturing of bandages and adhesive tapes.

Storage: It should be stored in tightly closed containers and protected from moisture.

Experiment 23

Preparation of Calcium Carbonate

Aim: To prepare and report the percentage yield of calcium carbonate from calcium chloride.

Requirements:

Calcium chloride, sodium carbonate, beakers, glass rod and funnels

Principle: Calcium carbonate is also called as precipitated chalk. It is prepared by the reaction between calcium chloride and sodium carbonate to give calcium carbonate and sodium chloride. Calcium carbonate is insoluble in water and hence it gets precipitated. Here 1 mole of calcium chloride reacts with 1 mole of sodium carbonate to gives 1 mole of calcium carbonate.

$$CaCl_2 . 2H_2O \quad or \quad CaCl_2 \;+\; Na_2CO_3 \longrightarrow CaCO_3 \downarrow \;+\; 2\ NaCl$$

$$147 \qquad\qquad 111 \qquad 106 \qquad\qquad\qquad 100 \qquad\quad 58.5$$

Procedure:

1. Dissolve the required amount (1.47 gm) of calcium chloride and dissolve in minimum amount of water.
2. Sodium carbonate solution is prepared by dissolving required amount of sample in minimum amount of water.
3. Heat both solutions up to the boiling point.
4. The boiling solution of calcium chloride is added to the boiling solution of sodium carbonate with continuous stirring.
5. The insoluble calcium carbonate is obtained is collected by filtration and dried.

Calculations:

Calculation of theoretical yield:

147 gm of calcium chloride yields ---------- > 100.1gm of calcium carbonate.

1.47 gm of calcium chloride yields ------------- > X gm.

$$X = \frac{1.47 \times 100.1}{147} = 1\ g$$

Theoretical yield = 1 gm.

Practical yield = -------------gm.

$$\text{Percentage yield} = \frac{\text{Practical yield}}{\text{Theoretical yield}} \times 100$$

$$= \frac{\text{gm}}{1} \times 100$$

$$= \text{--------}\%$$

Report: The product of calcium carbonate is prepared and submitted.

Practical yield	=	gm
Theoretical yield	=	gm
Percentage yield	=	%

Uses: Antacid, pharmaceutical aid (excipient)

Storage: Store in well-closed containers.

Experiment 24

Preparation of Magnesium Hydroxide

Aim: To prepare and report the percentage yield of magnesium hydroxide from magnesium sulphate.

Requirements:

Beakers, glass rod, funnel, light magnesium oxide and sodium hydroxide.

Principle: Magnesium hydroxide is prepared from magnesium sulphate which reacts with sodium hydroxide to yields magnesium hydroxide with the elimination of sodium sulphate. The product should be washed thoroughly to remove all sulphates. In this preparation magnesium oxide is added to get white and creamy consistent product. If magnesium oxide is not added , magnesium hydroxide would form a translucent, gelatinous aqueous suspension.

$$MgO \;+\; H_2O \longrightarrow Mg(OH)_2$$
$$40$$

$$(MgSO_4.7H_2O) \;\; or \;\; MgSO_4 + 2\,NaOH \longrightarrow Mg(OH)_2 \;+\; Na_2SO_4$$
$$246 \qquad\qquad 120 \qquad 40 \qquad\qquad\qquad 58.32 \qquad 142$$

Procedure:

1. Required quantity of light magnesium oxide is mixed with sodium hydroxide solution to get a cream. It is diluted with water.

2. The resulting suspension is poured in thin stream in to a solution of magnesium sulphate (prepared by dissolving 2.46 gm salt in minimum amount of water) with constant stirring.

3. The precipitate obtained is allowed to settle, the clear liquid is decanted off. The residue is transferred into a calico filter washed thoroughly with water until it is free from sulphate ions and dried.

Calculations:

Calculation of theoretical yield:

246.5 gm of magnesium sulphate yields ---------- > 58.3gm of magnesium hydroxide.

2.46 gm of magnesium sulphate yields ------------- > X gm.

$$X = \frac{2.46 \times 58.3}{246.5} = 0.58 \text{ g}$$

Theoretical yield = 0.58 gm

Practical yield = -------------gm.

$$\text{Percentage yield} = \frac{\text{Practical yield}}{\text{Theoretical yield}} \times 100$$

$$= \frac{\text{gm}}{0.58} \times 100$$

$$= \text{--------} \%$$

Report: The product of magnesium hydroxide is prepared and submitted.

Practical yield	=	gm
Theoretical yield	=	gm
Percentage yield	=	%

Uses: Antacid, Osmotic laxative.

Storage: Store in well-closed containers.

Experiment 25

Preparation of Calcium Lactate

Aim: To prepare and report the percentage yield of calcium lactate from calcium carbonate.

Requirements:

Beakers, glass rod, funnel, calcium carbonate, lactic acid and water.

Principle: Calcium lactate is prepared by the neutralization reaction between calcium carbonate and lactic acid. Here slight excess of calcium carbonate is added to the hot, dilute solution of lactic acid and boil the mixture until complete evaluation of carbon dioxide gas to gives calcium lactate. The main objective for boiling is to convert any anhydrides present in the mixture such as lactyl – lactic acid and lactide and complete the reaction. Here 1 mole of calcium lactate reacts with 1 mole of lactic acid to give 1 mole of calcium lactate.

$$CaCO_3 + 2\,CH_3\,CH(OH)\,COOH \longrightarrow [CH_3CH(OH)COO]_2Ca + CO_2 + H_2O$$

100	90	218
1.5g	1.8 g	2.18g
(0.015 mol)	(0.02 mol)	(0.01 mol)

Procedure:

1. Weigh accurately about 1.5 g (0.015 mol) (slight excess) of calcium carbonate.

2. Transfer the calcium carbonate powder in to a hot, dilute solution of lactic acid (1.8 g in water) and mix well.

3. Boil the above mixture for half an hour. Filter it in hot condition.

4. The colorless crystals of calcium lactate are obtained by evaporating the hot filtrate is collected, dried and weighed.

Calculations:

Calculation of theoretical yield:

100.1 gm of calcium carbonate yields --------- > 218.2 gm of calcium lactate.

1gm of calcium carbonate yields ------------ > X gm.

$$X = \frac{1 \times 218.2}{100.1}$$

Theoretical yield = 2.18 gm.

Practical yield = ------------gm.

$$\text{Percentage yield} = \frac{\text{Practical yield}}{\text{Theoretical yield}} \times 100$$

$$= \frac{\text{gm}}{0.6} \times 100$$

$$= \text{--------}\%$$

Report:

The sample of calcium lactate is prepared and submitted.

Practical yield	=	gm
Theoretical yield	=	gm
Percentage yield	=	%

Uses: Calcium replenisher.

Storage: Store in tightly closed containers.

3

Test for Purity

Introduction

Every pharmacopoeial monograph contains tests to ensure purity of the drugs. Several tests are included as qualitative and quantitative. Apart from identification tests that are qualitative, certain tests are necessary where assay methods cannot be established or needs to ensure for additional features eventhough the drug complies for qualitative and quantitative. Some of the tests that are unique are acid value, iodine value, saponification value, peroxide value, rancidity, unsaponifiable matter, ester value, ratio number, adsorbing power, defoaming activity, sodium alkyl sulphates, jelly strength, swelling power, threads per cm, weight per unit area, absorbency, fluorescence, congealing range, consistency, dynamic viscosity, setting properties, water absorption capacity, wool fat content etc.,

The current experiments illustrated are limited and are a sample of tests that are unique for a drug.

Experiment 26

Determination of Swelling Power of Bentonite

Aim: To determine the swelling power of bentonite by using apparent volume of sedimentation.

Requirements:

Bentonite, sodium lauryl sulphate (1%w/v solution), graduated measuring cylinder-100ml

Principle: The composition of bentonite is $Al_2O_3.6SiO_2.\chi H_2O$. It is insoluble in water but it shows remarkable swelling properties which forms a gel resembling like boiled starch when mixed with water. Due to these colloidal and absorptive properties, it is mainly used as a suspending agent in various pharmaceutical preparations. As per IP 1996, the apparent volume of the sediment at the bottom of the cylinder is not less than 24 ml.

Procedure:

1. Weigh accurately about 2gm of bentonite and divide into twenty equal portions.
2. Transfer 100ml of 1% w/v sodium lauryl sulphate solution into a graduated measuring cylinder (100ml capacity) about 3cm in diameter.
3. Add each portion of bentonite into the measuring cylinder at 2 min time intervals.
4. Allow each portion to settle before adding the next portion and allow to standing it for 2h.
5. The apparent volume of the sediment at the bottom of the cylinder should be noted.

Report: The swelling power of bentonite is ------   ml.

Experiment 27

Determination of Acid Neutralising Capacity of Aluminium Hydroxide Gel

Aim: To evaluate the acid neutralizing capacity of given sample by *in-vitro* method.

Requirements:

Antacid sample, 0.1M hydrochloric acid, sodium hydroxide solution (0.1M), pH meter.

Principle: Antacids are weak bases used to neutralize the excess gastric acid secretion associated with gastric and peptic ulcers. The acid neutralizing capacity of an antacid can be determined by two methods *in-vivo* and *in-vitro*. Many *in-vitro* techniques are reported. In the present method adding the antacid to a given amount of hydrochloric acid and measuring the amount of acid remaining and measuring the amount of acid consumed by the antacid to mimics the process occurring in stomach. Additional acid is added at given time intervals to mimic the continuing secretion of acid into the stomach. After one hour the content is titrated against sodium hydroxide and the acid remaining is determined. As per IP 1996, not more than 50.0 ml of 0.1 M NaOH is required.

In *in-vivo* evaluation of an antacid's acid neutralizing capacity is more difficult, because it involves removal of gastric contents at a particular time interval and measuring the pH.

Procedure:

1. Weigh accurately about 5gm of given sample and disperse in 100ml water. Heat the suspension up to 37° C.

2. Add 100.0 ml of 0.1M hydrochloric acid which is previously heated to 37° C.

3. Stirr it continuously, maintain the temperature at 37°C and measure the pH of the solution at time intervals of 10, 15 and 20 min and should be not less than 1.8, 2.3 and 3.0 respectively and at no time is more than 4.5.

4. To the above solution, add 10.0 ml of 0.5 M hydrochloric acid previously which is heated to 37° C, stirr continuously for 1 hour at 37°C and titrate with 0.1 M sodium hydroxide solution to a pH of 3.5.

Report: The amount of sodium hydroxide solution consumed is _____ ml. The acid neutralizing capacity of aluminium hydroxide gel is----- ml.

Experiment 28

Determination of Potassium Iodate in Potassium Iodide

Aim: To determine the presence of potassium iodate in the given sample of potassium iodide.

Requirements: Potassium iodide, dilute sulphuric acid and iodide free starch solution.

Principle: Impurity may be defined as any foreign substance present in the pharmaceuticals. Some of the impurities formed during the preparation of drugs/chemicals as intermediates. Some of these impurities may be carried into the final product also. In the preparation of potassium iodide, potassium iodate is formed as an intermediate which is liable and is present in the final product of potassium iodide. Hence IP has prescribed the test for iodate in potassium iodide. The presence of potassium iodate in potassium iodide can be detected by the formation of blue color with starch solution. The iodides of potassium iodide are oxidized to iodine by the oxidizing agent potassium iodate thereby the iodine reacts with starch solution and gives blue color.

$$KI \xrightarrow{KIO_3} I_2 \xrightarrow{Starch} Blue\ color$$

Procedure:

1. Weigh accurately about 0.5gm of potassium iodide (sample) and dissolve in 10ml carbon-dioxide free water.
2. Add 0.15ml/one drop of dilute sulphuric acid and add one drop of iodide free starch solution.
3. Observe the color of the solution.

Observation: No blue color is produced

Report: If no blue color is produced, indicates the amount of potassium iodate in potassium iodide is within the prescribed limit.

Experiment 29

Determination of Adsorption
Power in Heavy Kaolin

Aim: To determine and report the adsorption power of the given sample of heavy kaolin.

Requirements:

Methylene blue solution (0.003% w/v and 0.37% w/v), Heavy kaolin, test tubes, Centrifuger.

Principle: Kaolin adsorbs the blue color of methylene blue solution and the un-absorbed colour after dilution is compared with standard colour. Here known quantity of Kaolin is treated with known volume of known concentration of methylene blue. After centrifugation, a known volume of centrifugate, which is having blue colour, is diluted to 100 volumes with water. The diluted solution is compared with standard colour produced by 0.003% w/v solution of methylene blue. As per IP 1996, the test solution colour is not more intense than standard solution colour.

Procedure:

1. Weigh accurately 1.0 gm of heavy kaolin and transferred into a clean glass stoppered test tube.

2. Add 10 ml of 0.37 % w/v solution of methylene blue and shake well for 2 min.

3. Allow to settle for 2min. Centrifuge the mixture and dilute 1 volume of the solution to 100 ml with water.

4. Compare the intensity of color produced in the test solution with the standard methylene blue solution which is 0.003% w/v solution of methylene blue.

Observation & Report:

If the blue color produced in the test solution is less than that of the standard solution. The absorption power of heavy kaolin is within the prescribed limit of standards of I.P.

Experiment 30

Determination of Ferric Ion and Reducing Sugars in Ferrous Gluconate

Aim: To determine the ferric ion/reducing sugars present in the given sample of ferrous gluconate (or) to check the test for purity of the given sample of ferrous gluconate and report its compliance with the standards of I.P.

Requirements:

Ferrous gluconate sample, hydrochloric acid, potassium iodide, 0.1M sodium thiosulphate solution, starch solution, dilute ammonia solution, lead acetate paper, sodium carbonate solution, potassium cupric-tartarate solution, beakers, pipettes, volumetric flasks, burettes, conical flask and iodine flask.

Principle: Ferrous gluconate is prepared by the reaction between gluconic acid and ferrous sulphate. For this reaction, gluconic acid is obtained by the oxidation of glucose. So the reducing sugars may be present in the final products and ferrous sulphate containing any ferric ions means which may also present as an impurity in the final product. Hence, the I.P referred the test for purity of ferric ion/ reducing sugars in ferrous gluconate.

1. The presence of ferric ion as an impurity is determined by the iodometry method of titration.

2. Ferric ions oxidizes potassium iodide and liberates iodine, the liberated iodine is determined by titrating with sodium thiosulphate solution using starch solution as an indicator. End point is the disappearance of blue color.

$$Fe^{3+} + HI \ (KI + HCl) \longrightarrow I_2 \uparrow + Fe^{2+}$$

$$I_2 + 2\,Na_2S_2O_3 \longrightarrow 2\,NaI + Na_2S_4O_6$$

Sodium thiosulphate   Sodium tetrathionate

3. The presence of reducing sugar as an impurity is detected by using Fehling's test.

4. Reducing sugars (glucose, fructose etc), if present in the sample as an impurity reacts with Fehling's solution forming red color product.

Procedure:

For ferric ion:

1. Weight accurately about 5gm of ferrous gluconate sample and transfer into an iodine flask.

2. Add 100 ml of freshly boiled and cooled water and add 10ml of hydrochloric acid.
3. Transfer 3gm of potassium iodide into the above solution, shake well and keep it aside for 5minutes in dark.
4. During this reaction, the iodine is liberated which is titrated with 0.1M sodium thiosulphate solution using starch solution as an indicator. End point is the disappearance of blue color.
5. Blank determination also done. The difference between the two titre values gives the amount of iodine liberated by the ferric ion. Each ml of 0.1 M sodium thiosulphate is equivalent to 0.005585 g of ferric iron (1.0 %).

Procedure:

For reducing sugars:

1. Transfer 0.5gm of ferrous gluconate sample into a 100ml conical flask and dissolve in 10 ml of water.
2. Make the solution alkaline by the addition of dilute ammonia solution.
3. Pass hydrogen sulphide gas into the solution and keep it to stand for 30 min.
4. Collect the precipitate by filtration; wash thoroughly with each two quantities of 5ml of water.
5. Combine the filtrate and washings, acidity with dilute hydrochloric acid and add excess 2 ml of dilute hydrochloric acid.
6. Boil the solution until the vapors no longer darkens lead acetate paper.
7. Reduce the volume of the solution to 10ml by simple evaporation.
8. Cool the solution, add 10 ml of sodium carbonate solution, keep it aside for 5 minutes, filter it and make up the filtrate to 100 ml with water.
9. To the 5ml of filtrate, add 2 ml of potassium cupric tartarate solution (Fehling's solution) and boil for 1 min.
10. Observe the color of the solution.

Observation and Report:

For ferric ion: The difference between the two titre values is within the prescribed limit. The given sample complies with standards of I.P. and vice-versa.

For reducing sugars: If no red color precipitate is formed with Fehling's solution, the given sample complies with standards of I.P. and vice-versa.

4

Assay

Introduction

Assay is defined as the process of determining percentage purity of a test sample. This means, purity of the sample for every 100 g. In all the official pharmacopoeias, the bulk drug which means the pure form of the active drug that is used for manufacturing formulations is assayed for purity.

Now a days, pharmaceutical industries are concentrating on their drug for their purity in terms of establishing the impurity in addition to active drug. It is now mandatory to have the details of the impurity in terms of physical, chemical, pharmacological properties.

The percentage purity of a substance is determined based on chemical nature of the substance. The substance is assayed by one of the several methods like titrimetric, gravimetric, spectrometric etc., in broad sense.

As a titration, the sample may be assayed by one of the several methods like acid-base, redox, precipitation, complexometric, non-aqueous, conductimetric, potentiometric titrations.

As a spectroscopic, the sample can be assayed by ultraviolet-visible, flame photometric, atomic-absorption, phosphorescence, fluorescence, turbido-nephelometric, HPLC, GC etc., techniques.

Especially in quantitative determinations in assays, acid-base titrations are performed to substance that are basic-acid or a base or acid is liberated during the process of assay procedure. In a complexometric titration, a complex is made between the metallic samples with usual ligand ethylenediamine tetra-acetate disodium salt. In non-aqueous titration, a reaction with weakly basic (sodium citrate) or acidic (ethosuximide, hydrochlor thiazide, sulphafurazole, phenols) test substance is made to react with perchloric acid or potassium/ sodium/ lithium methoxide/ tetra butyl ammonium hydroxide in methanol respectively under no presence of water conditions.

For instance, halides like sodium chloride assayed by precipitation titration, zinc sulphate assayed by complexometric titration, barium sulphate assayed by gravimetric, sodium citrate by non-aqueous titration, sulphacetamide sodium by potentiometric titration, sodium ascorbate by redox titration, sodium bicarbonate by acid-base titration. As spectrometric assays, quinine sulphate by fluorescence, phenolphthalein by UV, microbiological by turbido-nephelometry, sodium in potassium chloride by atomic absorption spectrometry/flame photometry is used.

An assay is different from estimation. In an assay usually the active drug i.e., bulk drug is quantitatively analyzed for every 100 g. Where as in estimation, the drug present in the formulations (even though mentioned as assay) is determined and checked for the labeled value.

Experiment 31

Assay of Sodium Bicarbonate

Aim: To determine the percentage purity of given sodium bicarbonate.

Requirements: Sodium bicarbonate, 1 M hydrochloric acid, methyl orange indicator, burette, conical flasks, 20/25 ml bulb pipette, beakers, 100 ml volumetric flask, sodium carbonate.

Principle: Sodium bicarbonate IP 1996, contains not lessthan 99.0 percent and not morethan 101.0 percent of $NaHCO_3$. Sodium bicarbonate is basic in nature. Hence it is assayed by acid-base titration. Here standard 1 M hydrochloric acid is used. The prepared 1 M hydrochloric acid acts as an secondary standard after it is standardized by a primary standard sodium carbonate.

Here 1 mole of sodium bicarbonate reacts with 1 mole of hydrochloric acid giving sodium chloride, carbon dioxide and water.

$$NaHCO_3 + HCl \rightarrow NaCl + CO_2 + H_2O$$

$$2HCl + Na_2CO_3 \rightarrow 2NaCl + CO_2 + H_2O$$

Here methyl orange is used as indicator until colour changes.

Each ml of 1 M hydrochloric acid is equivalent to 0.08401 g of $NaHCO_3$.

Sodium bicarbonate is used as an alkaliser.

Procedure:

Titration: 1 M hydrochloric acid vs. sodium bicarbonate:

Weigh accurately 1.5 g of sample and dissolve in 50 ml of carbon dioxide free water and titrate with 1 M hydrochloric acid using 0.2 ml of methyl orange solution as indicator. A similar blank titration is carried out by omitting test sample and necessary correction in titer volume is made.

Observation:

Titration name: 1 M hydrochloric acid vs. sodium bicarbonate:

S. No.	Contents in the conical flasks	Initial burette reading a ml	Final burette Reading b ml	Volume consumed from burette a ~ b ml
1.				

Indicator: Methyl orange

Colour change:

Titration name: Blank titration: 1 M hydrochloric acid vs. blank:

S. No.	Contents in the conical flasks	Initial burette reading a ml	Final burette reading b ml	Volume consumed from burette a ~ b ml
1.				

Indicator: Methyl orange

Colour change:

Calculations:

Percentage purity of sodium bicarbonate =

Percentage purity =

$$\frac{\text{Titre value} \times \text{Actual molarity of HCl} \times \text{Eq.wt factor}}{\text{Weight of the sample taken} \times \text{Theorectical molarity of HCl}} \times 100$$

$$= \frac{\text{Volume of HCl} \times M_{HCl} \times \text{Eq. factor} \times 100}{1 \times \text{weight of sample(g)}}$$

Report: The percentage purity of given sodium bicarbonate =   %

Preparation of Reagents:

1. *1 M hydrochloric acid:* Solutions of any molarity x M may be prepared by diluting $85x$ ml of hydrochloric acid to 1000 ml with water.

2. *Methyl orange indicator:* Dissolve 0.1 g of methyl orange in 80 ml of water and add sufficient ethanol (95%) to produce 100 ml.

Standardisation of 1 M Hydrochloric Acid:

Weigh accurately about 10.6 g of sodium carbonate and transfer into a 100 ml volumetric flask. Dissolve in minimum water and make up the volume to 100 ml. Transfer 20.0 ml of the sodium carbonate solution into a conical flask and titrate the solution with hydrochloric acid using methyl red solution as indicator until the solution becomes faintly pink. Heat the solution to boiling, cool and continue the titration. Heat again to boiling and titrate further as necessary until the faint pink colour is no longer affected by continued boiling. (Perform a blank titration if necessary).

Each ml of 1 M hydrochloric acid is equivalent to 0.05299 g of Na_2CO_3.

Titration Name: 1 M hydrochloric acid vs. std. sodium carbonate:

S. No.	Contents in the conical flasks	Initial burette reading a ml	Final burette reading b ml	Volume consumed from burette a ~ b ml	Concurrent value
1.					

Indicator: Methyl orange

Colour change:

Calculation of molarity of sodium carbonate:

106 g of sodium carbonate in 1000 ml gives→1 M sodium carbonate solution.

10.6 g of sodium carbonate in 100 ml gives → 1 M sodium carbonate solution.

X (actually weighed) g of sodium carbonate in 100 ml gives → ? M sodium carbonate solution.

$$M_1 = \frac{\text{weight taken}}{\text{weight to be taken}} \times \text{original Molarity}$$

Molarity of sodium carbonate solution prepared = X/ 10.6 × 1 = M_1 M

Hence molarity of sodium carbonate solution prepared = M_1 M

Molarity of Hydrochloric acid $M_2 = M_1 V_1 n_2 / V_2 n_1$

$$= M$$

where,

    M_1 = Molarity of sodium carbonate solution

    V_1 = Volume of sodium carbonate solution pipetted

    n_1 = Number of moles of sodium carbonate

    M_2 = Molarity of hydrochloric acid

    V_2 = Volume of hydrochloric acid consumed

    n_2 = Number of moles of hydrochloric acid

Experiment 32

Assay of Magnesium Sulphate

Aim: To determine the percentage purity of given magnesium sulphate.

Requirements: Magnesium sulphate, 0.05M di-sodium edetate, strong ammonia-ammonium chloride solution, mordant black II indicator, conical flasks, 10 ml measuring cylinder, 20/25 ml bulb pipette, beakers, 100 ml volumetric flask, di-sodium edetate.

Principle: Magnesium sulphate IP 1996, contains not lessthan 99.0 percent and not morethan 100.5 percent of $MgSO_4$, calculated with reference to the dried substance.

Magnesium sulphate is assayed by complexo-metric titration using di-sodium ethylene diamine tetra acetate.

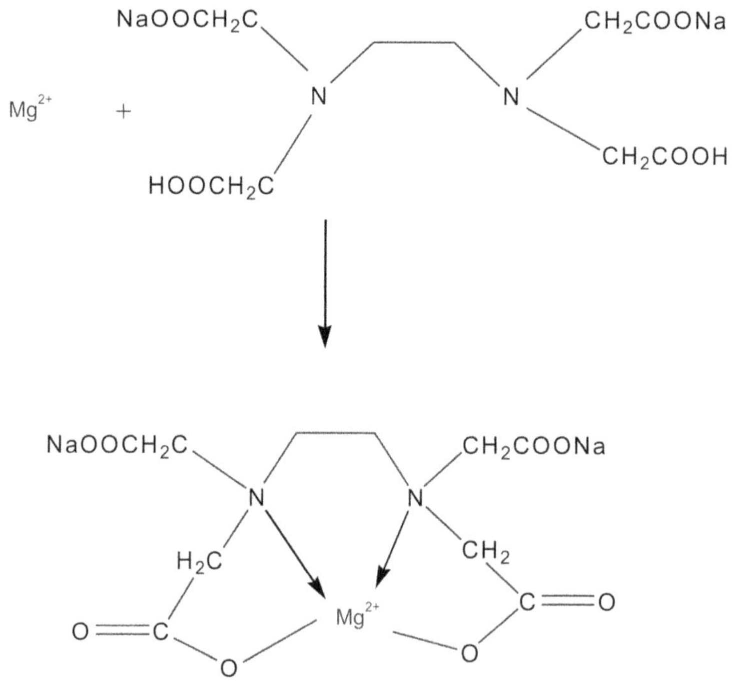

Here, ammonia-ammonium chloride is used as buffer to maintain pH of the solution so as to maintain stability of the complex. Here mordant black II comprising of 1 part of eriochrome black T dispersed in 99 parts of sodium chloride is used as indicator until colour changes from wine red to blue.

Here, disodium edetate, since possess most characters of primary standard, a solution can be prepared by known weight and judging its molarity from weight transferred dissolving in a known accurate volume of water.

A blank titration omitting test substance is carried and necessary titer volume corrections are made.

Each ml of 0.05M disodium edetate is equivalent to 0.00602g of $MgSO_4$.

As a secondary standard solution, disodium edetate is standardized using primary standard zinc and dissolving with hydrochloric acid.

Magnesium sulphate is also called as epsom salt. It is used as osmotic laxative, electrolyte replenisher.

Procedure:

Weigh accurately 0.3 g and dissolve in 50 ml of water, add 10 ml of strong ammonia-ammonium chloride solution and titrate with 0.05 M disodium edetate, using 0.1 g of mordant black II indicator until blue colour is obtained.

Observation:

Titration name: 0.05 M disodium edetate vs magnesium sulphate

S. No.	Contents in the conical flasks	Initial burette reading a ml	Final burette reading b ml	Volume consumed from burette a ~ b ml
1.				

Indicator: Mordant black II indicator

Colour change:

Titration name : Blank titration: 0.05M di sodium edetate vs. blank:

S. No.	Contents in the conical flasks	Initial burette reading a ml	Final burette reading b ml	Volume consumed from burette a ~ b ml
1.				

Indicator: Mordant black II indicator

Colour change:

Calculations:

Percentage purity of magnesium sulphate

$$= \frac{\text{Volume of disodium EDTA} \times M_{EDTA} \times \text{Eq. factor} \times 100}{0.05 \times \text{weight of sample(g)}}$$

Report: The percentage purity of given magnesium sulphate =   %

Preparation of Reagents:

1. *0.05 M disodium edetate:* Solutions of any molarity x M may be prepared by dissolving 372.2x g of disodium edetate in sufficient water to produce 1000 ml.

2. *Mordant black II indicator:* A mixture of 1 part of eriochrome black T and 99 parts of sodium chloride.

3. *Strong ammonia-ammonia chloride solution:* Dissolve 67.5 g of ammonium chloride in 740 ml of strong ammonia solution and add sufficient water to produce 1000 ml.

Calculation of Molarity of Disodium Edetate:

372.2 g of disodium edetate in 1000 ml gives → 1 M disodium edetate solution.

37.22 g of disodium edetate in 1000 ml gives → 0.1 M disodium edetate solution.

18.61g of disodium edetate in 1000 ml gives → 0.05 M disodium edetate solution.

X (actually weighed) g of disodium edetate in 1000 ml gives → ? M disodium edetate solution.

Molarity of disodium edetate solution prepared = X/ 18.61 × 0.05 = M_1 M

Hence molarity of disodium edetate solution prepared = M_1 M

Experiment 33

Assay of Barium Sulphate

Aim: To determine the percentage purity of given barium sulphate.

Requirements: Barium sulphate, sodium carbonate, potassium carbonate, hydrochloric acid, 10% w/v potassium dichromate, furnace, platinum/ silica crucible, 40% w/v ammonium acetate, urea.

Principle: Barium sulphate IP 1996, contains not less than 97.5 percent and not more than 100.5 percent of $BaSO_4$.

Barium sulphate is assayed by gravimetric method which is not usually like a titration.   Here a known quantity of sample is processed and made to react with a specific reagent i.e. potassium dichromate to get a precipitate of barium chromate. The quantitatively produced barium chromate is weighed and the quantity of barium sulphate to give the precipitate is back calculated and finally the percentage.

Here, barium sulphate is first treated with sodium/potassium carbonate to convert into insoluble barium carbonate and soluble sodium/potassium sulphate. The precipitated barium carbonate is thoroughly washed and made free from sulphate impurities. The precipitate is then made to react with hydrochloric acid so as to convert to soluble form of barium chloride. The resultant is filtered and the filterate containing soluble form of barium chloride is made to react with excess potassium dichromate to convert into insoluble form of barium chromate.

$$BaSO_4 + Na_2CO_3 \; \rightarrow BaCO_3 \downarrow + Na_2SO_4$$

$$BaCO_3 + HCl \rightarrow BaCl_2 + H_2O + CO_2$$

$$BaCl_2 + K_2Cr_2O_7 \rightarrow BaCr_2O_7 + KCl$$

Each g of the residue is equivalent to 0.9213 g of $BaSO_4$.

Barium sulphate is used as a diagnostic agent i.e., as radio-opaque medium for gastrointestinal tract. As suspensions, are called as barium meal.

Procedure:

Weigh accurately about 0.60 g in a platinum crucible, add 5 g of sodium carbonate and 5 g of potassium carbonate and mix. Heat to 1000 °C and maintain at this temperature for 15 minutes. Allow to cool and suspend the residue in 150 ml of water. Wash the crucible with 2 ml of acetic acid and add to the suspension. Cool in ice and filter by decantation, transferring as little of the solid matter as possible to the filter. Wash the residue with successive quantities of a 2% w/v solution of sodium carbonate until the washings are free from sulphate and discard the washings. Add 5 ml of dilute hydrochloric acid to the filter and wash through into the vessel containing the bulk of the solid matter with water. Add 5 ml of hydrochloric acid and dilute to 100 ml with water. Add 10 ml of a 40% w/v solution of ammonium acetate, 25 ml of a 10% w/v solution of potassium dichromate and 10 g of urea. Cover, digest in an oven at 80 °C to 85 °C for 16 hours and filter while still hot through a sintered-glass filter (porosity No. 4), washing the precipitate initially with a 0.5 % w/v solution of potassium dichromate and finally with 2 ml of water. Dry to constant weight at 105 °C, weigh, calculate and report.

Observation:

Weight of barium chromate obtained = x g

Calculations:

0.9213 g of barium sulphate gives → 1 g of barium chromate

Theoretically 0.6 g of barium sulphate gives → 0.6/0.9213 × 1

$$= y \text{ g of barium chromate}$$

If y g of barium chromate from 0.6 g of barium sulphate indicates → 100 %

x g of barium chromate obtained from 0.6 of sample indicates → x/y × 100 = %

Report: The percentage purity of given barium sulphate =   %

Preparation of Reagents:

1. *0.5% w/v potassium dichromate solution*: A 0.5% w/v solution of potassium dichromate in water.

2. *10% w/v potassium dichromate solution:* A 10% w/v solution of potassium dichromate in water.

3. *2% w/v sodium carbonate solution:* A 2% w/v solution of sodium carbonate in water.

4. *40% w/v ammonium acetate solution:* A 40% w/v solution of ammonium acetate in water.

5. *Dilute hydrochloric acid:* Approximately 10% w/w of hydrochloric acid in water.

Experiment 34

Assay of Sodium Chloride

Aim: To determine the percentage purity of sodium chloride.

Requirements: Sodium chloride, 0.1 M silver nitrate, 2 M nitric acid, dibutyl phthalate, 0.1 M ammonium thiocyanate, ferric ammonium sulphate solution, burettes, conical flasks, 25/50 ml bulb pipette, 100 ml volumetric flask, silver nitrate.

Principle: Sodium chloride IP 1996, contains not less than 99.0 percent and not more than 100.5 percent of NaCl, calculated with reference to the dried substance.

Halides are usually assayed by argentometry titration i.e., using silver nitrate. Among the Mohr's, Volhard's, Fajan's methods, one is used.

Here, to the sample solution an excess known concentration of silver nitrate solution is added and the excess un-reacted silver nitrate is estimated by a back titration using standard ammonium thiocyanate solution. Here, dibutyl phthalate is added to form a protective layer on the silver chloride precipitate, to prevent silver chloride reacting with ammonium thiocyanate and not to interfere in the back titration. Here ferric ammonium sulphate (ferric alum) is used as indicator.

$$NaCl + AgNO_3 \rightarrow AgCl \downarrow + NaNO_3$$

$$excess$$

$$AgNO_3 + NH_4SCN \rightarrow AgSCN \downarrow + NH_4NO_3$$
un-reacted
(not from AgCl)

$$NH_4SCN + Fe^{3+} \rightarrow Fe(SCN)_3 + NH_4^{+}$$
$$red$$

Each ml of 0.1 M silver nitrate is equivalent to 0.005844 g of NaCl.

A back titration is one, estimation of un-reacted after addition of excess reagent.

A blank titration is one in which titration is carried out similar to test compound but omitting the test compound. The objective of blank titration is to minimize error caused during titration by the impurities, if any present.

Sodium chloride is a pharmaceutical aid as a tonicity agent, fluid and electrolyte replenisher.

Procedure:

Weigh accurately about 0.1 g and dissolve in 50 ml of water in a glass-stoppered flask. Add 50.0 ml of 0.1 M silver nitrate, 5 ml of 2 M nitric acid and 2 ml of dibutyl phthalate, shake well and titrate with 0.1M ammonium thiocyanate using 2 ml of ferric ammonium sulphate solution as indicator, until the colour become reddish yellow. (Perform a back titration omitting sample)

Observation:

Titration name:

0.1 M ammonium thiocyanate vs. silver nitrate (sodium chloride)

S. No.	Contents in the conical flasks	Initial burette reading a ml	Final burette reading b ml	Volume consumed from burette a ~ b ml
1.				

Indicator: Ferric ammonium sulphate

Colour change:

Titration name:

Back Titration: 0.1 M ammonium thiocyanate vs. silver nitrate

S. No.	Contents in the conical flasks	Initial burette reading a ml	Final burette reading b ml	Volume consumed from burette a ~ b ml
1.				

Indicator: Ferric ammonium sulphate

Colour change:

Calculations:

Percentage purity of sodium chloride

$$= \frac{\text{Volume of NH}_4\text{SCN} \times \text{M}_{\text{NH}_4\text{SCN}} \times \text{Eq. factor} \times 100}{0.1 \times \text{weight of sample(g)}}$$

Report: The percentage purity of given sodium chloride =   %

Preparation of reagents:

1. *0.1 M ammonium thiocyanate:* Solutions of any molarity xM may be prepared by dissolving $76.12x$ g in sufficient water to produce 1000 ml.

2. *0.1 M silver nitrate solution:* Solutions of any molarity *x* M may be prepared by dissolving 170*x* g of silver nitrate in sufficient water to produce 1000 ml.

3. *2 M nitric acid:* Solutions of any molarity *x* M may be prepared by diluting 63*x* ml of nitric acid to 1000 ml with water.

4. *Ferric ammonium sulphate solution:* An 8.0 % w/v solution of ferric ammonium sulphate in water.

Standardization of 0.1 M ammonium thiocyanate:

Weigh accurately about 1.6987 g of silver nitrate (primary standard) and transfer into a 100 ml volumetric flask. Dissolve in minimum water and make up the volume to 100 ml. Transfer 20.0 ml of the silver nitrate solution into a conical flask, dilute with 50 ml water, add 2 ml of nitric acid and 2 ml of ferric ammonium sulphate solution and titrate with the ammonium thiocyanate solution until the solution becomes red-brown colour. (Perform a blank titration omitting silver nitrate)

Each ml of 0.1 M silver nitrate is equivalent to 0.007612 g of NH_4SCN.

Titration Name: 0.1 M ammonium thiocyanate vs. std. silver nitrate:

S. No.	Contents in the conical flasks	Initial burette reading a ml	Final burette reading b ml	Volume consumed from burette a ~ b ml	Concurrent value
1.					

Indicator: Ferric ammonium sulphate

Colour change:

Titration Name: BlankTitration: 0.1 M ammonium thiocyanate vs. blank solution:

S. No.	Contents in the conical flasks	Initial burette Reading a ml	Final burette Reading b ml	Volume consumed from burette a ~ b ml	Concurrent value
1.					

Indicator: Ferric ammonium sulphate

Colour change:

Calculation of Molarity of Silver Nitrate:

169.87 g of silver nitrate in 1000 ml gives → 1 M silver nitrate solution.

16.987 g of silver nitrate in 1000 ml gives → 0.1 M silver nitrate solution.

1.6987 g of silver nitrate in 100 ml gives $\rightarrow$ 0.1 M silver nitrate solution.

X (actually weighed) g of silver nitrate in 100 ml gives $\rightarrow$?

$$\text{M silver nitrate solution.}$$

Molarity of silver nitrate solution prepared $= (X/\ 1.6987) \times 0.1 =\ M_1$ M

Hence molarity of silver nitrate solution prepared $=\ M_1$ M

Molarity of ammonium thiocyanate soution $M_2 = M_1\ V_1\ n_2\ /\ V_2\ n_1$

$$=\quad M$$

where,

M_1 = Molarity of silver nitrate solution

V_1 = Volume of silver nitrate solution pipetted

n_1 = Number of moles of silver nitrate

M_2 = Molarity of ammonium thiocyanate

V_2 = Volume of ammonium thiocyanate consumed (corrected volume)

n_2 = Number of moles of ammonium thiocyanate

Experiment 35

Assay of Sodium Citrate

Aim: To determine the percentage purity of sodium citrate.

Requirements: Sodium citrate, anhydrous glacial acetic acid, 0.1 M perchloric acid, 1-napthol benzein solution, acetic anhydride, crystal violet solution, conical flask, 20/25 ml conical flasks, 100 ml volumetric flask, burette, potassium hydrogen phthalate.

Principle: Sodium citrate IP 1996, contains not less than 99.0 percent and not more than 101.0 percent of $C_6H_5Na_3O_7$, calculated with reference to the anhydrous substance.

Sodium citrate is assayed by non-aqueous titration. Usually, weak acids or weak bases are assayed by non-aqueous titration. The word itself indicates that the titration is carried out in strictly water free conditions. If water is present in the titration, hydroxyl group of water competes with weakly basic substance on titration with standard perchloric acid.

Here, solvents glacial acetic acid, acetic anhydride are used in non-aqueous titration and 1-naphthol benze in solution as indicator.

$$3\ CH_3COOH + 3\ HClO_4 \rightarrow 3\ CH_3COOH_2^+ + 3\ ClO_4^-$$

$$C_6H_5Na_3O_7 + 3\ CH_3COOH \rightarrow C_6H_8O_7 + 3\ CH_3COO^-$$

$$3\ CH_3COOH_2^+ + 3\ CH_3COO^- \rightarrow 6\ CH_3COOH$$

$$C_6H_5Na_3O_7 + 3\ HClO_4 \rightarrow C_6H_8O_7 + 3\ ClO_4^-$$

Each ml of 0.1 M perchloric acid is equivalent to 0.008602 g of $C_6H_5Na_3O_7$.

Secondary standard perchloric acid is standardized by primary standard potassium hydrogen phthalate.

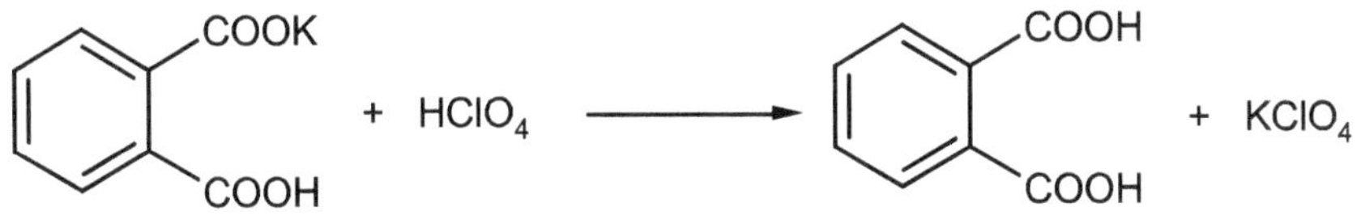

Sodium citrate is also called as tri-sodium citrate. It is used as systemic alkalinizing agent.

Procedure:

Weigh accurately about 0.15 g and dissolve in 20 ml of anhydrous glacial acetic acid, warming to about 50 °C. Allow to cool and titrate with 0.1 M perchloric acid using 0.25 ml of 1-naphthol benzein solution as indicator.

Observation:

Titration name: Perchloric acid vs. sodium citrate

S. No.	Contents in the conical flasks	Initial burette reading a ml	Final burette reading b ml	Volume consumed from burette a ~ b ml
1.				

Indicator: 1-naphthol benzein solution

Colour change:

Titration name: Perchloric acid vs. blank

S. No.	Contents in the conical flasks	Initial burette reading a ml	Final burette reading b ml	Volume consumed from burette a ~ b ml
1.				

Indicator: 1-naphthol benzein solution

Colour change:

Calculations:

Percentage purity of sodium citrate

$$= \frac{\text{Volume of } HClO_4 \times M_{HClO_4} \times \text{Eq. factor} \times 100}{0.1 \times \text{weight of sample(g)}}$$

Report: The percentage purity of given sodium citrate =   %

Preparation of Reagents:

1. *0.1 M perchloric acid:* Mix 8.5 ml of perchloric acid with 500 ml of anhydrous glacial acetic acid and 25 ml of acetic anhydride, cool and add anhydrous glacial acetic acid to produce 1000 ml.

2. *1-napthol benzein solution:* A 0.2 % w/v solution of 1-naphthol benzein in anhydrous glacial acetic acid.

3. *Crystal violet solution:* A 0.5 % w/v solution of crystal violet in anhydrous glacial acetic acid.

Standardisation of 0.1 M Perchloric Acid:

Weigh accurately about 2.0422 g of potassium hydrogen phthalate (primary standard) and transfer into a 100 ml volumetric flask. Dissolve in minimum glacial acetic acid and make up the volume to 100 ml with glacial acetic acid. Transfer 20.0 ml of the potassium hydrogen phthalate solution into a conical flask, add 0.1 ml of crystal violet solution and titrate with the perchloric acid solution until the violet colour solution becomes emerald-green colour. (Perform a blank titration omitting potassium hydrogen phthalate).

Titration Name:

0.1 M perchloric acid vs. std. potassium hydrogen phthalate:

S. No.	Contents in the conical flasks	Initial burette reading a ml	Final burette reading b ml	Volume consumed from burette a ~ b ml	Concurrent value
1.					

Indicator: Crystal violet solution

Colour change:

Titration Name: BlankTitration: 0.1 M perchloric acid vs. blank solution:

S. No.	Contents in the conical flasks	Initial burette reading a ml	Final burette reading b ml	Volume consumed from burette a ~ b ml	Concurrent value
1.					

Indicator: Crystal violet solution.

Colour change:

Calculation of Molarity of Perchloric Acid:

204.22 g of potassium hydrogen phthalate in 1000 ml gives→1 M potassium hydrogen phthalate solution.

20.4220 g of potassium hydrogen phthalate in 1000 ml gives → 0.1 M potassium hydrogen phthalate solution.

2.0422 g of potassium hydrogen phthalate in 100 ml gives $\rightarrow$ 0.1 M potassium hydrogen phthalate solution.

X (actually weighed) g of potassium hydrogen phthalate in 100 ml gives $\rightarrow$? M potassium hydrogen phthalate solution.

Molarity of potassium hydrogen phthalate solution prepared

$$= (X/\,2.0422) \times 0.1 = M_1 \; M$$

Hence molarity of potassium hydrogen phthalate solution prepared $= M_1$ M

Molarity of Perchloric acid soution $M_2 = M_1\, V_1\, n_2\, /\, V_2\, n_1$

$$= M$$

where,

M_1 = Molarity of potassium hydrogen phthalate solution

V_1 = Volume of potassium hydrogen phthalate solution pipetted

n_1 = Number of moles of potassium hydrogen phthalate

M_2 = Molarity of perchloric acid

V_2 = Volume of perchloric acid consumed (corrected volume)

n_2 = Number of moles of perchloric acid.

Experiment 36

Assay of Hydrogen Peroxide

Aim: To determine the percentage purity of hydrogen peroxide solution (20 vol).

Requirements: Hydrogen peroxide solution (20 vol), 1 M sulphuric acid, 0.02 M potassium permanganate, conical flask, 20/25 ml conical flasks, 100 ml volumetric flask, burette, 1 ml bulb pipette, oxalic acid.

Principle: Hydrogen peroxide solution (20 vol) IP 1996, contains not less than 5.0 percent w/v and not more than 7.0 percent w/v of H_2O_2, corresponding to about 20 times its volume of available oxygen.

Hydrogen peroxide solution (20 vol) is assayed by redox titration. A redox titration involves oxidation, reduction reaction. Hydrogen peroxide is a strong oxidizing agent. But, in presence of potassium permanganate, hydrogen peroxide eventhough oxidizing agent acts as reducing agent. Hence, in this titration potassium permanganate acts as strong oxidizing agent and hydrogen peroxide as reducing agent. Here the titration is carried out in presence of acid so as to dissolve all the products formed in the titration.

Here potassium permanganate acts as self indicator. At the end point the colour of the solution is purple.

$$2\ KMnO_4 + 5\ H_2O_2 + 3\ H_2SO_4 \rightarrow 2\ MnSO_4 + K_2SO_4 + 5\ O_2 \uparrow + 8\ H_2O$$

Each ml of 0.02 M potassium permanganate is equivalent to 0.001701 g of H_2O_2.

Here, secondary standard potassium permanganate solution is standardized by primary standard either oxalic acid or sodium oxalate. Indian Pharmacopoeia 1996, uses iodometry method of standardization of potassium permanganate.

Hydrogen peroxide solution (20 vol) is an aqueous solution of hydrogen peroxide. It may contain a suitable stabilizing agent.

Hydrogen peroxide solution (20 vol) is also called as hydrogen peroxide solution (6%) or dilute hydrogen peroxide solution. It is used as antiseptic, deodorant.

Procedure:

Transfer 1.0 ml of hydrogen peroxide solution (20 vol) into a conical flask and add 20 ml of 1 M sulphuric acid and titrate with 0.02 M potassium permanganate solution until colour changes from colour less to purple.

Observation:

Titration name:

Potassium permanganate vs. hydrogen peroxide solution (20 vol)

S. No.	Contents in the conical flasks	Initial burette reading a ml	Final burette reading b ml	Volume consumed from burette a ~ b ml
1.				

Indicator: Potassium permanganate (self indicator)

Colour change:

Titration name: Potassium permanganate vs. blank

S. No.	Contents in the conical flasks	Initial burette reading a ml	Final burette reading b ml	Volume consumed from burette a ~ b ml
1.				

Indicator: Potassium permanganate (self indicator)

Colour change:

Calculations:

Percentage purity of hydrogen peroxide solution (20 vol)

$$= \frac{\text{Volume of KMnO}_4 \times \text{M}_{\text{KMnO}_4} \times \text{Eq. factor} \times 100}{0.1 \times 1}$$

Report:

The percentage purity of given hydrogen peroxide solution (20 vol) =   %

Preparation of Reagents:

1. *0.02 M Potassium permanganate:* Dissolve 3.2 g of potassium permanganate in 1000 ml of water, heat on a water bath for 1 hour, allow to stand for 2 days and filter through glass wool. Store in light-resistant container.

2. *1 M sulphuric acid:* Solutions of any molarity x M may be prepared by carefully adding $54x$ ml of sulphuric acid to an equal volume of water and diluting to 1000 ml with water.

Standardisation of 0.02 M Potassium Permanganate:

Weigh accurately about 0.252 g of oxalic acid (primary standard) and transfer into a 100 ml volumetric flask. Dissolve in minimum water and make up the volume to 100 ml with water. Transfer 20.0 ml of the oxalic acid solution into a conical flask, add 20 ml of 1 M sulphuric acid and boil the solution to about 80-90 °C and titrate with the potassium permanganate solution until the solution becomes colour less to purple. (Perform a blank titration omitting oxalic acid).

Titration Name: 0.02 M potassium permanganate vs. std. oxalic acid:

S. No.	Contents in the conical flasks	Initial burette reading a ml	Final burette reading b ml	Volume consumed from burette a ~ b ml	Concurrent value
1.					

Indicator: Potassium permanganate (self indicator)

Colour change:

Titration Name: BlankTitration: 0.02 M potassium permanganate vs. blank solution:

S. No.	Contents in the conical flasks	Initial burette reading a ml	Final burette reading b ml	Volume consumed from burette a ~ b ml	Concurrent value
1.					

Indicator: Potassium permanganate (self indicator)

Colour change:

Calculation of Molarity of Potassium Permanganate:

126 g of oxalic acid in 1000 ml gives →1 M oxalic acid solution.

12.6 g of oxalic acid in 100 ml gives → 1 M oxalic acid solution.

1.26 g of oxalic acid in 100 ml gives → 0.1 M oxalic acid solution.

0.126 g of oxalic acid in 100 ml gives → 0.01 M oxalic acid solution.

0.252 g of oxalic acid in 100 ml gives → 0.02 M oxalic acid solution.

X (actually weighed) g of oxalic acid in 100 ml gives →?

M oxalic acid solution.

Molarity of oxalic acid solution prepared = $(X/\,0.252) \times 0.02 = \ M_1 \ $ M

Hence molarity of oxalic acid solution prepared = M_1 M

Molarity of potassium permanganate solution $M_2 = M_1 V_1 n_2 / V_2 n_1$

$$= \quad M$$

where,

M_1 = Molarity of oxalic acid solution

V_1 = Volume of oxalic acid solution pipetted

n_1 = Number of moles of oxalic acid

M_2 = Molarity of potassium permanganate

V_2 = Volume of potassium permanganate consumed (corrected volume)

n_2 = Number of moles of potassium permanganate

Experiment 37

Assay of Chlorinated Lime

Aim: To determine the assay of the given sample of chlorinated lime.

Requirements:

Chlorinated lime, acetic acid, potassium iodide 0.1 M sodium thiosulphate solution, starch mucilage, beakers. burette, conical flasks, bulb pipettes (20 ml and 25 ml), volumetric flask (100 ml).

Principle: It is assayed by iodometry method of titration (also called redox titration) to find out the "available chlorine".

In this assay the substance is treated with acetic acid in presence of excess of potassium iodide and titrated with sodium thiosulphate, using starch mucilage as an indicator. End point is the disappearance of blue color.

In this assay when the substance is reacted with acetic acid in presence of excess of potassium iodide, available chlorine is liberated from chlorinated lime and it displaces equal amount of iodine from potassium iodide. The liberated iodine is determined by titrating with N/10 sodium thiosulphate using starch mucilage as an indicator. End point is the disappearance of blue colour. During this titration iodine is reduced to sodium iodide and sodium thiosulphate is oxidized to sodium tetrathionate. As the oxidation and reduction takes place simultaneously this is called Redox titration. The chemical reactions of this assay are shown below.

$$Ca(OCl)Cl + 2\ CH_3COOH \longrightarrow (CH_3COO)_2Ca + HOCl + HCl$$
(Chlorinated
  lime)

$$HOCl + HCl \rightleftharpoons Cl_2 + H_2O$$

$$Cl_2 + 2KI \longrightarrow I_2 + 2\ KCl$$

$$I_2 + 2\ Na_2S_2O_3 \longrightarrow 2\ NaI + Na_2S_4O_6$$
$$\text{Sodium} \qquad\qquad\qquad \text{Sodium tetrathionate}$$
$$\text{thiosulphate}$$

Procedure:

Triturate 4 gm of chlorinated lime with small quantities of water and dilute to 1000 ml with water and shake thoroughly. Mix 100 ml of the resulting suspension with a solution containing 3 gm of potassium iodide in 100 ml of water, acidify with 5 ml of 6M acetic acid and titrate the liberated iodine with 0.1M sodium thiosulphate, using starch mucilage as an indicator. End point is the disappearance of blue color.

Each ml of 0.1 M sodium thiosulphate is equivalent to 0.003545 gm of chlorine.

Chlorinated Lime Vs 0.1M Sodium Thiosulphate

S. No.	Content of conical flask.	Burette reading in (ml).		Concordant value in (ml).	Indicator (End point)
		Initial volume	Final volume		
					Starch mucilage (Disappearance of blue color).

Blank Determination:

S. No.	Content of conical flask.	Burette reading in (ml).		Concordant value in (ml).	Indicator (End point)
		Initial volume	Final volume		
					Starch mucilage (Disappearance of blue color).

Calculations:

Calculation of molarity of 0.1 M sodium thiosulphate solution:

Molarity of 0.1 M sodium thiosulphate solution is calculated by using the following formula

Actual molarity of 0.1 M sodium thiosulphate solution =

$$\frac{\text{Titre value} \times \text{equivalent weight factor}}{\text{Weight of the sample taken}}$$

Calculation of percentage purity of chlorinated lime:

The percentage purity of chlorinated lime is determined by using the following formula.

Percentage purity =

$$\frac{\text{Titre value} \times \text{actual molarity of sodium thiosulphate} \times \text{Eq. wt factor}}{\text{Weight of the sample taken} \times \text{Theoretical molarity of sodium thiosulphate}} \times 100$$

Report: According to I.P, It contains not less than 30% w/w of available chlorine.

The percentage purity of the given sample of hydrogen peroxide is found to be ------.%

Preparation of Reagents:

1. **0.1M sodium thiosulphate solution:** Dissolve 25 gm of sodium thiosulphate and 0.2 gm of sodium carbonate in carbon dioxide free water and dilute to 1000 ml with water.
2. **Starch mucilage:** Triturate 0.5 gm of starch or soluble starch with 5 ml of water with continuous stirring to produce 100 ml with water. Boil for few minutes and filter.
3. **Starch solution:** Triturate 1gm of soluble starch with 5 ml of water with continuous stirring to produce 100 ml with boiling water containing 10 mg of mercuric iodide.

Standardization of 0.1 M Sodium Thiosulphate Solution:

In this assay, 0.1 M sodium thiosulphate solution acts as a secondary standard which is standardized by titrating against a primary standard potassium bromate. The procedure for the standardization is as follows.

Dissolve 0.2 gm of potassium bromate in 250 ml of water. To the 50 ml of the solution add 2 gm of potassium iodide and 3 ml of 2 M hydrochloric acid and titrate with the sodium thiosulphate solution using starch solution as an indicator, which is added to the end of the titration. End point is the disappearance of blue color

Each ml of 0.1 M sodium thiosulphate is equivalent to 0.002784 gm of $KBrO_3$.

Potassium Bromate Vs 0.1M Sodium Thiosulphate

S. No.	Content of conical flask.	Burette reading in (ml).		Concordant value in (ml).	Indicator (End point)
		Initial volume	Final volume		
					Starch solution (Disappearance of blue color).

Note: An official sample contains about 30% Cl_2.

Experiment 38

Assay of Iodine

Aim: To determine the percentage purity of the given sample of iodine.

Requirements:

Chlorinated lime, acetic acid, potassium iodide 0.1M sodium thiosulphate solution, starch mucilage, beakers. Burette, conical flasks, bulb pipettes (20 ml and 25 ml), volumetric flask (100 ml).

It is assayed by Iodimetry method of titration (also called Redox titration).

In this assay the substance is dissolved in a solution of Pottasium iodide in an iodine flask. The solution is made acidic by treating with acetic acid and titrated with N/10 sodium thiosulphate using starch mucilage as an indicator. End point is the disappearance of blue colour. During this titration iodine is reduced to sodium iodide and sodium thiosulphate is oxidised to sodium tetrathionate. As the oxidation and reduction takes place simultaneously this is called Redox titration. The chemical reactions of this assay are shown below.

$$I_2 + 2Na_2S_2O_3 \longrightarrow 2\,NaI + Na_2S_4O_6$$

Sodium   Sodium tetrathionate
thiosulphate

Each ml of 0.1 M sodium thiosulphate is equivalent to 0.01269 g of Iodine.

As per IP 1996, Iodine contains not less than 99.5 percent and not more than 100.5 percent of Iodine.

Procedure:

Weigh accurately about 0.2 g, transfer to a conical flask containing 1 g of potassium iodide and 2 ml of water, 1 ml of acetic acid , dissolve completely and add 50 ml of water. Titrate with 0.1 M sodium thiosulphate using starch solution as an indicator. End point is the disappearance of blue color.

Iodine Vs 0.1M Sodium Thiosulphate

S. No.	Content of conical flask.	Burette reading in (ml).		Concordant value in (ml).	Indicator (End point)
		Initial volume	Final volume		
					Starch solution (Disappearance of blue color).

Blank Determination:

S. No.	Content of conical flask.	Burette reading in (ml).		Concordant value in (ml).	Indicator (End point)
		Initial volume	Final volume		
					Starch solution (Disappearance of blue color).

Calculations:

Calculation of molarity of 0.1 M sodium thiosulphate solution:

Molarity of 0.1 M sodium thiosulphate solution is calculated by using the following formula

Actual molarity of 0.1 M sodium thiosulphate solution

$$= \frac{\text{Titre value} \times \text{equivalent weight factor}}{\text{Weight of the sample taken}}$$

Calculation of Percentage Purity of Iodine:

The percentage purity of chlorinated lime is determined by using the following formula.

Percentage purity =

$$\frac{\text{Titre value} \times \text{actual molarity of sodium thiosulphate} \times \text{Eq. wt factor}}{\text{Weight of the sample taken} \times \text{original molarity of sodium thiosulphate}} \times 100$$

Report: The percentage purity of the given sample of Iodine is found to be ------ %.

Standardization of Reagents:

Standardization of 0.1 M Sodium Thiosulphate Solution:

In this assay, 0.1 M sodium thiosulphate solution acts as a secondary standard which is standardized by titrating against a primary standard potassium bromate. The procedure for the standardization is as follows.

Dissolve 0.2 gm of potassium bromate in 250 ml of water. To the 50 ml of the solution add 2 gm of potassium iodide and 3 ml of 2 M hydrochloric acid and titrate with the sodium thiosulphate solution using starch solution as an indicator, which is added to the end of the titration. End point is the disappearance of blue color.

Each ml of 0.1 M sodium thiosulphate is equivalent to 0.002784 gm of $KBrO_3$.

Potassium Bromate Vs 0.1M Sodium Thiosulphate

S. No.	Content of conical flask.	Burette reading in (ml).		Concordant value in (ml).	Indicator (End point)
		Initial volume	**Final volume**		
					Starch solution (Disappearance of blue color).

Preparation of Reagents:

1. **0.1M sodium thiosulphate solution:** Dissolve 25 gm of sodium thiosulphate and 0.2 gm of sodium carbonate in carbon dioxide free water and dilute to 1000 ml with water.

2. **Starch mucilage:** Triturate 0.5 gm of starch or soluble starch with 5 ml of water with continuous stirring to produce 100 ml with water. Boil for few minutes and filter.

3. **Starch solution:** Triturate 1 gm of soluble starch with 5 ml of water with continuous stirring to produce 100 ml with boiling water containing 10 mg of mercuric iodide.

Experiment 39

Assay of Ferrous Sulphate

Aim: To determine the assay of the given sample of ferrous sulphate.

Requirements:

Ferrous sulphate (sample), sodium bicarbonate, sulphuric acid, 0.1 M ceric ammonium nitrate, ferroin solution, beakers. burette, conical flasks, bulb pipettes (20 ml and 25 ml), volumetric flask (100 ml).

Principle: It is assayed by ceriometry method of titration (also called redox titration).

In this assay sample is dissolved in water and 1M sulphuric acid and titrated a with 0.1M ceric ammonium nitrate using ferroin sulphate as indicator. End point is the disappearance of red colour.

$$Fe^{2+} \longrightarrow Fe^{3+} + e$$
$$Ce^{4+} + e \longrightarrow Ce^{3+}$$
$$NaAsO_2 + 2H_2O \longrightarrow NaH_2AsO_4 + 2H^+ + 4e$$
$$4[Ce^{4+} + e \longrightarrow Ce^{3+}]$$

As per IP 1996, ferrous sulphate contains not less than 98.0 percent and not more than 105.0 percent of $FeSO_4 . 7H_2O$.

Procedure:

Dissolve 2.5 gm of sodium bicarbonate in a mixture of 150 ml of water and 10 ml of sulphuric acid. When effervescence ceases, add about 0.5 gm of ferrous sulphate. Shake gently to dissolve and titrate with 0.1M ceric ammonium nitrate, using 0.1 ml of ferroin solution as indicator End point is the disappearance of red color.

Each ml of 0.1 M ceric ammonium nitrate is equivalent to 0.02780 gm of $FeSO_4 . 7H_2O$.

Ferrous Sulphate Vs 0.1 M Ceric Ammonium Nitrate

S. No.	Content of conical flask.	Burette reading in (ml).		Concordant value in (ml).	Indicator (End point)
		Initial volume	Final volume		
					Ferroin (disappearance of red color).

Blank Determination:

S. No.	Content of conical flask.	Burette reading in (ml).		Concordant value in (ml).	Indicator (End point)
		Initial volume	Final volume		
					Ferroin (disappearance of red color).

Calculations:

Calculation of molarity of 0.1 M ceric ammonium nitrate solution:

Molarity of 0.1 M ceric ammonium nitrate solution is calculated by using the following formula

Actual molarity of 0.1 M sodium thiosulphate solution

$$= \frac{\text{Titre value} \times \text{equivalent weight factor}}{\text{Weight of the sample taken}}$$

Calculation of percentage purity

The percentage purity of ferrous sulphate is determined by using the following formula.

Percentage purity =

$$\frac{\text{Titre value} \times \text{actual molarity of ceric ammonium nitrate} \times \text{Eq. wt factor}}{\text{Weight of the sample taken} \times \text{Theoretical molarity of ceric ammonium nitrate}} \times 100$$

Report: The percentage purity of the given sample of ferrous sulphate is found be ------%

Preparation of Reagents:

1. **0.1 M ceric ammonium nitrate solution:** Dissolve 54.820gm of ceric ammonium nitrate in 56 ml of sulphuric acid and shake well for 2 minutes, carefully add five successive quantities, each 100 ml of water, shake well after each addition. Dilute the clear solution to 1000 ml with water. After 10 days standardize the solution.

2. **Ferroin solution:** Dissolve 0.7 gm of ferrous sulphate and 1.5 gm of 1, 10 – phenanthroline hydrochloride in 70 ml of water and make up to produce 100 ml with water.

3. **Osmic acid solution:** A 1% w/v solution of osmic acid in water. (Osmic acid is osmium tetraoxide : OsO_4)

Standardization of 0.1 M Ceric Ammonium Nitrate Solution:

In this assay, 0.1 M ceric ammonium nitrate solution acts as a secondary standard which is standardized by titrating against a primary standard arsenic trioxide. The procedure for the standardization is as follows.

Weigh accurately about 0.2 gm of arsenic trioxide, previously dried at 105 ^{0} C for 1 hour and tranfered to a 500 ml conical flask. Wash down the inner walls of the flask with 25 ml of 8 % w/v sodium hydroxide solution, swirl to dissolve. Add 100 ml of water and mix. To this add 30 ml of dilute sulphuric acid and 0.15 ml of osmic acid solution, 0.1 ml of Ferroin sulphate solution and slowly titrate with ceric ammonium nitrate solution until the color change from pink to very pale blue, adding the titrant slowly towards the endpoint.

Each ml of 0.1 M ceric ammonium nitrate is equivalent to 0.004946 gm of As_2O_3.

Arsenic Trioxide Vs 0.1M Ceric Ammonium Nitrate

S. No.	Content of conical flask.	Burette reading in (ml).		Concordant value in (ml).	Indicator (End point)
		Initial volume	Final volume		
					Ferroin sulphate (pink to very pale blue).

Experiment 40

Assay of Heavy Magnesium Oxide

Aim: To perform the assay of the given sample of heavy magnesium oxide

Requirements:

Hydrochloric acid, ammonia- ammonium chloride solution,0.05 M EDTA solution, mordant black II indicator, beakers, burette, conical flasks, bulb pipettes (20 ml and 25 ml), volumetric flask (100 ml).

Principle: It is assayed by Complexometry method of (Direct) titration.

In this assay the substance is dissolved in hydrochloric acid, to this ammonia-ammonium chloride solution is added as buffer solution and it is then titrated against 0.05M disodium Ethylene Diamine Tetra Acetate (EDTA) using mordant black II mixture as an indicator.

End point is the appearance of blue colour.

In this assay magnesium ions of heavy magnesium oxide reacts with disodium EDTA, whereby the complexation takes place. As the magnesium ions forms complex with disodium EDTA in this assay, it is called as complexometry method of titration. The chemical reactions of this assay are shown below.

$$MgO \text{ (In soluble in water)} + 2HCl \longrightarrow MgCl_2 \text{ (Soluble in water)} + H_2O$$

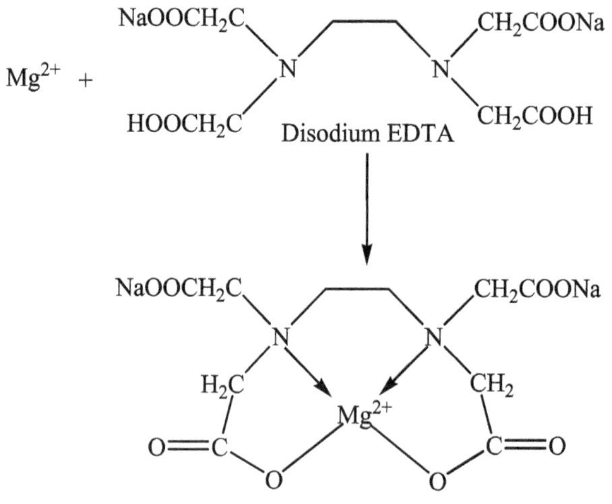

Disodium EDTA

Magnesium-EDTA Complex

Each ml of 0.05 M disodium edetate is equivalent to 0.002015 g of MgO.

As per IP 2014, heavy magnesium oxide contains not less than 98.0 percent and not more than 100.5 percent of MgO, calculated with reference to the substance ignited at 900 °C.

Procedure: Weigh accurately about 0.35 gm of heavy magnesium oxide, dissolve it in 10 ml of 2M hydrochloric acid, and dilute with water to 100.0 ml. To the 10.0 ml of solution add 5 ml of strong ammonia-ammonium chloride solution and titrate with 0.05M disodium edetate solution using about 0.05 g (50 mg) of mordant black II mixture as an indicator. End point is the disappearance of pink color.

Heavy Magnesium Oxide Vs 0.05 M Disodium EDTA

S. No.	Content of conical flask.	Burette reading in (ml).		Concordant value in (ml).	Indicator (End point)
		Initial volume	Final volume		
					Mordant black II mixture (the disappearance of pink color).

Blank Determination:

S. No.	Content of conical flask.	Burette reading in (ml).		Concordant value in (ml).	Indicator (End point)
		Initial volume	Final volume		
					Mordant black II mixture (the disappearance of pink color).

Calculations:

Calculation of Percentage Purity

The percentage purity of heavy magnesium oxide is determined by using the following formula.

Percentage purity =

$$\frac{\text{Titre value} \times \text{actual molarity of disodium EDTA} \times \text{Eq. wt factor}}{\text{Weight of the sample taken} \times \text{Theoretical molarity of disodium EDTA}} \times 100$$

Report: The percentage purity of the given sample of disodium EDTA is found to be ------ %.

Preparation of Reagents:

1. **0.05 M Disodium EDTA:** Dissolve 37.2 gm of disodium edetate in 1000 ml of water.

2. **Mordant black II indicator solution:** Triturate 1 part of eriochrome black T in 99 parts of sodium chloride.

3. **Strong ammonia – ammonium chloride solution:** Dissolve 67. 5 g of ammonium chloride in 740 ml of strong ammonia solution and add sufficient water to produce 1000 ml.

Standardization of 0.05 M Disodium EDTA Solution:

In this assay, 0.05 M disodium EDTA solution acts as a secondary standard which is standardized by titrating against a primary standard granulated zinc. The procedure for the standardization is as follows.

Weigh accurately about 0.4 gm of granulated zinc, dissolve it in 6 ml of dilute hydrochloric acid by gentle heating and add 0.1 ml of bromine water. Excess bromine is removed by boiling, cool and add sufficient amount of water to produce 100.0 ml. Pipette 10.0 ml of the resulting solution in to a conical flask and neutralize with 2 M sodium hydroxide. Dilute to 150 ml with water, add sufficient amount of ammonia buffer to make pH of the solution to 10 to dissolve the precipitate and add 5 ml in excess. Add 50 mg of mordant black II mixture and titrate with the 0.05M disodium edetate solution until the solution turns green.

Each ml of 0.05 M disodium EDTA is equivalent to 0.00654 gm of Zn.

Granulated Zinc Vs 0.05 M Disodium EDTA

S. No.	Content of conical flask.	Burette reading in (ml).		Concordant value in (ml).	Indicator (End point)
		Initial volume	Final volume		
					Mordant black II mixture (appearance of pink color).

Calculation of molarity of 0.05 M disodium EDTA solution:

Molarity of 0.05 M disodium EDTA solution is calculated by using the following formula

Actual molarity of 0.05 M disodium EDTA solution

$$= \frac{\text{Titre value} \times \text{equivalent weight factor}}{\text{Weight of the sample taken}}$$

5

Identification of Anions and Cations

Anions

1. Acetates

Test	Observation	Inference
1. Transfer a small quantity of test substance into a test tube and add equal quantity of oxalic acid. Heat. $CH_3COONa + C_2H_2O_4 \rightarrow CH_3COOH + C_2HNaO_4$	Acidic vapours with odour of acetic acid	Acetates
2. Transfer 1g of the substance into a test tube and add 1ml of sulphuric acid and 3 ml of ethanol (95%). Warm. $2CH_3COONa + H_2SO_4 + 2C_2H_5OH \rightarrow 2CH_3COOC_2H_5 + Na_2SO_4 + 2H_2O$	Sweet odour, smell of ethyl acetate	Acetates
3. Transfer 30 mg of the substance into a test tube and add 3ml water. Dissolve. Add 0.25 ml of lanthanum nitrate solution, 0.1 ml of 0.1M iodine and 0.05 ml of dil. NH_3 solution. Heat carefully to boiling. (Lanthanum acetate adsorbed by iodine)	Blue precipitate	Acetates

2. Benzoates

Test	Observation	Inference
1. Transfer 1ml of 10% neutral solution of the substance. Add 0.5 ml of $FeCl_3$ test solution. $3C_6H_5COONa + 2Fe^{3+} + 3H_2O \rightarrow$ $(C_6H_5COO)_3Fe.Fe(OH)_3\downarrow + 3H^+$	Dull yellow precipitate	Benzoates
2. Transfer 0.2 g of the substance into a test tube and add 0.3 ml of sulphuric acid. Warm gently at the bottom of the test tube. $2C_6H_5COONa + H_2SO_4 \rightarrow$ $C_6H_5COOH + Na_2SO_4$	White sublimate on the inner wall of the tube.	Benzoates

3. Bicarbonates

Test	Observation	Inference
1. Transfer small quantity of substance into a test tube. Add 3 ml water. Dissolve. Add $MgSO_4$ solution. $Mg^{2+} + 2\ NaHCO_3 \rightarrow$ $MgCO_3 + H_2O + CO_2 + 2\ Na^+$	No precipitate, but white precipitate on boiling.	Bicarbonate (distinction from carbonates)
2. Transfer 0.1 g of the substance into a test tube and add 2 ml water. Add 2 ml of 2 M acetic acid. Close the tube immediately using a stopper fitted with a glass tube bent at two right-angles. Heat gently and collect the gas in 5 ml of barium hydroxide solution. $NaHCO_3 + CH_3COOH \rightarrow$ $CH_3COONa + H_2O + CO_2 \uparrow$ $CO_2 \uparrow + Ba(OH)_2 \rightarrow BaCO_3\downarrow + H_2O$ $BaCO_3 + 2HCl \rightarrow BaCl_2 + H_2O + CO_2$	A white precipitate dissolves in excess dil. HCl	Bicarbonates

4. Bromides

Test	Observation	Inference
1. Transfer small quantity of the substance into a test tube and add 2 ml water. Add 2 M HNO_3 until solution is acidic. Add 1 ml of 0.1 M $AgNO_3$. Shake. $NaBr+AgNO_3 \rightarrow AgBr + NaNO_3$	Curdy pale yellow precipitate sparingly soluble in 1.5 ml 10 M NH_3.	Bromide
2. Transfer small quantity of substance into a test tube and add 2 ml water. Add 1 ml of chlorine solution. Bromine is evolved which is soluble in 2-3 drops of chloroform forming a reddish solution. To the aqueous solution containing the liberated bromine add phenol solution. $2NaBr+Cl_2 \rightarrow Br_2+2Cl^-$ $3Br_2+C_6H_5OH \rightarrow C_6H_2Br_3+3HBr$ *Note*: As iodides interfere the test, add lead dioxide to the sample solution and boil to remove iodine as vapours.	White precipitate	Bromide

5. Carbonates

Test	Observation	Inference
1. Transfer 0.1 g of the substance into a test tube and add 2 ml water. Add 2 ml 2 M acetic acid and close the tube immediately using a stopper fitted with a glass tube bent at two right-angles. Heat gently. Collect the gas in 5 ml of 0.1 M barium hydroxide solution. $Na_2CO_3+2CH_3COOH \rightarrow 2CH_3COONa+H_2O+CO_2\uparrow$ $CO_2\uparrow+Ba(OH)_2 \rightarrow BaCO_3\downarrow+H_2O$ $BaCO_3\downarrow + 2HCl \rightarrow BaCl_2 + H_2O + CO_2\uparrow$	White precipitate dissolves in excess dil.HCl	Carbonates
2. Transfer small quantities of the substance into a test tube and add 2 ml water. Add solution of $MgSO_4$. $Na_2CO_3+MgSO_4 \rightarrow MgCO_3+Na_2SO_4$	White precipitate	Carbonates distinct from bicarbonate

6. Chlorides

Test	Observation	Inference
1. Transfer small quantity of the substance into a test tube. Add 2 ml water. Acidify with dil.HNO$_3$. Add 0.5 ml of silver nitrate solution. Shake and allow to stand. $NaCl+AgNO_3 \rightarrow AgCl+NaNO_3$ $AgCl+2NH_3 \rightarrow [Ag(NH_3)_2]^+ +Cl^-$ $[Ag(NH_3)_2]^+ +Cl^- +2H^+ \rightarrow AgCl+2NH_4^+$	Curdy white precipitate insoluble in dil. HNO$_3$, but soluble in dil.NH$_3$	Chlorides
2. Transfer small quantity of the substance into a test tube. Add 0.2 g of potassium dichromate and 1 ml H$_2$SO$_4$. Place a filter paper strip moistened with 0.1 ml of diphenyl carbazide solution over the mouth of the test tube. $4 NaCl+K_2Cr_2O_7+3H_2SO_4 \rightarrow$ $2CrO_2Cl_2+3H_2O$	Paper turns violet-red	Chlorides

7. Citrates

Test	Observation	Inference
1. Transfer small quantity of the substance into a test tube and dissolve in water. Neutralize the solution and add calcium chloride solution. $2C_6H_5O_7Na_3+3CaCl_2 \rightarrow Ca_3(C_6H_5O_7)_2$	No precipitate, but on boiling white precipitate. Soluble in 6 M acetic acid	Citrates
2. Transfer small quantity of the substance into a test tube and add 2ml water. Add 0.5 ml H$_2$SO$_4$ and 3 ml KMnO$_4$ solution. Warm until colour of solution is discharged and add 0.5 ml of 10% sodium nitroprusside in 1M H$_2$SO$_4$ and 4 g of sulphamic acid. The solution is made alkaline with strong ammonia solution until sulphamic acid has dissolved. Add excess ammonia solution.	Violet colour turns to violet-blue	Citrates

8. Iodides

Test	Observation	Inference
1. Transfer small quantity of substance into a test tube and add 2 ml water. Add dil.HNO_3 and 0.5 ml silver nitrate solution. Shake and allow to stand. $NaI+AgNO_3 \rightarrow AgI+NaNO_3$	Pale yellow precipitate insoluble in dil. NH_3	Iodides
2. Transfer small quantity of substance into a test tube and add 2 ml water. Add 0.5 ml of 1 M H_2SO_4, 0.15 ml of potassium di chromate solution, 2 ml water and 2 ml chloroform. Shake and allow to stand. $6NaI+K_2Cr_2O_7+7H_2SO_4 \rightarrow$ $3I_2+3Na_2SO_4+Cr_2(SO_4)_3+K_2SO_4+7H_2O$	Violet or violet-red colour observed in chloroform layer	Iodides
3. Transfer small quantity of substance into a test tube and add 2 ml water. Add 0.5 ml of mercuric chloride solution. $2NaI+HgCl_2 \rightarrow HgI_2+2NaCl$ $HgI_2+2KI \rightarrow [HgI_4]^{2-}$	Dark red precipitate slightly soluble in excess of the reagent and very soluble in excess of potassium iodide solution	Iodides

9. Lactates

Test	Observation	Inference
1. Transfer 5 mg of substance into a test tube and add 5 ml water. Add 1 ml of bromine water and 0.5 ml of 1 M sulphuric acid. Heat on a water bath, stirring occasionally with a glass rod until the colour discharged. Add 4 g of ammonium sulphate, mix and add dropwise without mixing 0.2 ml of 10% sodium nitroprusside solution in 1M sulphuric acid. Without mixing, add 1 ml of strong ammonia solution and allow to stand for 30 minutes.	Dark green ring appears at the interface of the two liquids	Lactates

10.   Nitrates

Test	Observation	Inference
1. Transfer 15 mg of the substance into a test tube and add 0.5 ml of water. Add cautiously 1 ml of sulphuric acid, mix and cool. Incline the tube and carefully add, without mixing, 0.5 ml of ferrous sulphate solution. $2NaNO_3+4H_2SO_4+6FeSO_4\rightarrow$ $6Fe^{3+}+2NO\uparrow+4(SO_4)^{2-}+4H_2O$ $Fe^{2+}+NO\rightarrow[Fe(NO)]^{2+}$	A brown colour at the interface of two liquids.	Nitrates
2. Transfer 0.1 ml of nitro benzene and 0.2 ml of sulphuric acid and mix. Add 10 mg of test substance. Allow to stand 5 minutes and cool in ice. Add 5ml of water and 5 ml of sodium hydroxide solution. Add 5 ml of acetone, shake and allow to stand.	Intense violet colour in the upper layer	Nitrates

11.   Salicylates

Test	Observation	Inference
1. Transfer 1ml of 10% w/v of neutral solution into a test tube. Add 0.5 ml of ferric chloride solution. $C_7H_5O_3Na+FeCl_3\rightarrow complex$	A violet colour persists after addition of acetic acid	Salicylates
2. Transfer 0.5 g of the substance into a test Tube. Add 10 ml of water. Add 2 ml of bromine Solution. $C_7H_5O_3Na+Br_2\rightarrow C_7H_5O_3Br+NaBr$	A cream-coloured precipitate formed.	Salicylates

12. Silicates

Test	Observation	Inference
1. Transfer 200 mg of the test substance into a platinum crucible and add 10 mg of sodium fluoride and a few drops of sulphuric acid. Mix to form a slurry. Cover the crucible with a thin transparent plate of plastic under which a drop of water is suspended and warm gently. $Na_2SiO_3+4NaF+3H_2SO_4\rightarrow3Na_2SO_4+SiF_4+3H_2O$ $3SiF_4+2H_2O\rightarrow SiO_2\downarrow+2[SiF_6]^{2-}+4H^+$	A white ring is formed around the drop of water.	Silicates

13.   Sulphates

Test		Observation	Inference
1.	Transfer 50 mg of the test substance into a test tube and add 5 ml water. Add 1 ml of dilute hydrochloric acid and 1 ml of barium chloride solution. $Na_2SO_4+BaCl_2 \rightarrow BaSO_4\downarrow+2NaCl$	White precipitate	Sulphates
2.	Add 0.1 ml of iodine solution to the suspension obtained in the above test. The suspension remains yellow (distinction from sulphites and dithionites) but is decolorized by adding dropwise, stannous chloride solution (distinction from iodates). Boil the mixture. $PbSO_4 + 2\ CH_3COONH_4 \rightarrow$ $(CH_3COO)_2Pb + (NH_4)_2SO_4$	No coloured precipitate	Sulphates
3.	Transfer 50 mg of the test substance into a test tube and add 5 ml of water. Add 2 ml of lead acetate solution. $Na_2SO_4+(CH_3COO)_2Pb \rightarrow PbSO_4\downarrow+2CH_3COONa$	White precipitate soluble in ammonium acetate and in sodium hydroxide solution.	Sulphates

14.   Tartarates

Test	Observation	Inference
1. Transfer 10 mg of the test substance into a test tube and add 2 drops of sulphuric acid. Warm. $C_4H_4O_6Na_2+H_2SO_4 \rightarrow C_4H_6O_6+Na_2SO_4$	Charring with carbon monoxide. on burning gives blue flame.	Tartarates
2. Transfer 20 mg of the test substance into a test tube and add 1 ml of water. Add 0.05 ml of a 1 % w/v solution of ferrous sulphate and 0.05 ml of hydrogen peroxide (10 vol). After transient yellow colour produced, add 2M sodium hydroxide dropwise.	Intense blue colour	Tartarates
3. Transfer 2 mg of tartaric acid and dissolve in 0.5 ml of water. Heat on a water bath for 5 to 10 minutes with 0.1 ml of 10% w/v solution of potassium bromide, 0.1 ml of 2% w/v solution of resorcinol and 3 ml of sulphuric acid. $C_4H_4O_6Na_2+H_2SO_4 \rightarrow CH_2OH.CHO$ glycollic aldehyde $C_6H_4(OH)_2+CH_2OH.CHO \rightarrow$ $CH_2OH.CH[C_6H_3(OH)_2]_2$	Dark blue colour changing to red when cooled and poured into water.	Tartarates

15. Thiosulphates

1.	Transfer 0.1 g of the test substance into a test tube and add 5 ml of water. Add 2 ml of hydrochloric acid. $Na_2S_2O_3+2HCl \rightarrow S\downarrow+SO_2+H_2O$	White precipitate which turns yellow and sulphur dioxide recognizable odour.	Thiosulphate.
2.	Transfer 0.1 g of the test substance into a test tube and add 5 ml of water. Add 2 ml of ferric chloride test solution. $Na_2S_2O_3+FeCl_3 \rightarrow [Fe(S_2O_3)_2]^-$ $[Fe(S_2O_3)_2]^-+Fe^{3+} \rightarrow 2Fe^{2+}+S_4O_6^{2-}$ $2S_2O_3^{2-}+2Fe^{3+} \rightarrow S_4O_6^{2-}+2Fe^{2+}$	Dark violet colour quickly disappears.	Thiosulphate.
3.	Transfer 10 mg of test substance into a test tube and add 1 ml of water. Add iodine solution. $I_2+2Na_2S_2O_3 \rightarrow 2NaI+Na_2S_4O_6$	Decolourized solution do not give tests for sulphates.	Thiosulphate.
4.	Transfer 10 mg of test substance into a test tube and add 1 ml of water. Add bromine solution.	Decolourized solution give tests for sulphates.	Thiosulphate.

Cations

1. Aluminium

1.	Transfer 20 mg of the test substance into a test tube and add 2 ml of water. Add 0.5 ml of 2 M hydrochloric acid and 0.5 ml of thioacetamide reagent. No precipitate is produced. Add drop wise 2 M sodium hydroxide solution. $AlCl_3 + NaOH \rightarrow Al(OH)_3$ $Al(OH)_3 + OH^- \rightarrow [Al(OH)_4]^-$	Gelatinous white precipitate, redissolve on addition of further 2M sodium hydroxide. reappears on addition of ammonium chloride solution.	Aluminium
2.	Transfer 20 mg of the test substance into a test tube and add 5 ml of water. add 5 drops of ammonium acetate solution, 5 drops of 0.1% w/v solution of mordant blue 3. $Al^{3+} + ligand \rightarrow complex$	Intense purple colour	Aluminium
3.	Transfer 20 mg of the test substance into a test tube and add 5 ml of water. Add dilute ammonia solution. A faint precipitate is produced. Then add 0.25 ml of freshly prepared 0.05 % w/v solution of quinalizarin in a 1 % w/v solution of sodium hydroxide. Heat to boiling, cool, and acidify with an excess of acetic acid. Formation of ammonium quinalizarinate	Reddish violet colour	Aluminium

2. Ammonium

1. Transfer 10 mg of the test substance into a test tube and add 1 ml of sodium hydroxide solution. Heat. $NH_4Cl+NaOH \rightarrow NH_3\uparrow+NaCl+H_2O$	Ammonia vapours, turns red litmus to blue.	Ammonium
2. Transfer 100 mg of the test substance into a test tube and add 1 ml water. Add 0.2 mg of light magnesium oxide. Pass a current of air through the mixture and direct the gas that is evolved to just beneath the surface of a mixture of 1 ml of 0.1 M hydrochloric acid and 0.05 ml of methyl red solution. $3NH_4^{+}+[Co(NO_2)_6]^{3-} \rightarrow (NH_4)_3[Co(NO_2)_6]$	Colour of solution changes to yellow. Yellow precipitate is produced on addition of 1 ml of freshly prepared 10% w/v solution of sodium cobaltinitrite.	Ammonium

3. Antimony

1. Transfer 0.5 mg of sodium potassium tartarate into a test tube and add 10 ml of water. Add 10 mg of test substance and heat gently until dissolve. Allow to cool. To 2 ml of the solution add sodium sulphide solution dropwise. $SbCl_3+3H_2S \rightarrow Sb_2S_3+6H^{+}$	Reddish orange precipitate. Dissolves on adding dilute sodium hydroxide solution.	Antimony

4. Arsenic

1. Transfer 10 mg of the test substance into a test tube and add 0.5 ml of water. Add equal volume of hypophosphorus reagent. Heat on a water bath.	Brown precipitate	Arsenic

5. Barium

1.	Transfer 50 mg of the test substance on to a watch glass. Add two drops of hydrochloric acid. Introduce the paste in the non-luminous flame of the burner. Observe the colour of the flame. $BaSO_4+2HCl \rightarrow BaCl_2+H_2SO_4$	Yellowish green colour. Appears blue through a green glass.	Barium
2.	Transfer 20 mg of the test substance into a tube and add 1 ml of water. Add 1 ml dilute hydrochloric acid and 0.5 ml of dilute sulphuric acid. $BaCl_2+H_2SO_4 \rightarrow BaSO_4\downarrow+2HCl$	White precipitate. Insoluble in nitric acid.	Barium

6. Bismuth

1.	Transfer 0.5 mg of the test substance into a test tube and add 10 ml of 2 M hydrochloric acid. Heat to boiling for 1 minute. Cool and filter, if necessary. To 1 ml of the filterate add 20 ml of water. $2BiCl_3+3H_2S \rightarrow Bi_2S_3+6HCl$	White or slight yellow precipitate. turns brown on addition of sodium sulphide solution.	Bismuth
2.	Transfer 50 mg of test substance into a test tube and add 10 ml of 2 M nitric acid. Heat to boiling for 1 minute. Allow to cool and filter, if necessary. To 5 ml of the filterate add 2 ml of a 10 %w/v solution of thiourea.	Orange-yellow colour or precipitate. No decolourisation on addition of 4 ml of 2.5%w/v solution of sodium fluoride.	Bismuth

7. Calcium

1.	Transfer 20 mg of the test substance into a test tube and add 5 ml 5 M acetic acid. Add 0.5 ml of potassium ferrocyanide solution. The solution remains clear. Add about 50 mg of ammonium chloride. $CaCl_2+K_2[Fe(CN)_6]\rightarrow K_2Ca[Fe(CN)_6]$	White crystalline precipitate.	Calcium
2.	Transfer 20 mg of the test substance in to a test tube and add 1 ml water. Dissolve with few drops of acid if not dissolved. Add 0.2 ml of 2 % w/v solution of ammonium oxalate. $CaCl_2+(COONH_4)_2\rightarrow(COO)_2Ca$ $(COO)_2Ca+HCl\rightarrow(COOH)_2 +CaCl_2$	White precipitate. Sparingly soluble in dilute acetic acid. Soluble in hydrochloric acid.	Calcium
3.	Transfer 20 mg of the test substance into a test tube and add few drops of dilute hydrochloric acid to dissolve. Neutralize excess acid with dilute sodium hydroxide solution. Add 5 ml of ammonium carbonate solution. $CaCl_2+(NH_4)_2CO_3\rightarrow CaCO_3+2NH_4Cl$	White precipitate. Sparingly soluble in ammonium chloride on boiling and cooling.	Calcium

8. Ferric

1.	Transfer 10 mg of the test substance into a test tube and add 1 ml water. Add 1 ml of potassium ferro cyanide solution. $4Fe^{3+}+3[Fe(CN)_6]^{4-}{\rightarrow}Fe_4[Fe(CN)_6]_3$	Intense blue precipitate. Insoluble in dilute hydro chloric acid	Ferric
2.	Transfer 0.1 mg of the test substance into a test tube and add few drops of 2 M hydrochloric acid and few drops of ammonium thiocyanate solution. $Fe^{3+}+3SCN^{-}{\rightarrow}Fe(SCN)_3$	Blood red colour.	Ferric
3.	To one portion of above test solution add 1 ml ether. Shake and allow to stand.	Pink colour in ether layer.	Ferric
4.	To second portion of above test solution add few drops of 0.2 M mercuric chloride. $2Fe(SCN)_3+3Hg^{2+}{\rightarrow}2Fe^{3+}+3Hg(SCN)_2$	Red colour disappears	Ferric
5.	Transfer 0.1 mg of the test substance into a test tube and add 0.5 ml water to dissolve. Add acetic acid until solution is strongly acidic. Add 2 ml of 0.2 %w/v solution of 8-hydroxy-7-iodoquinoline-5-sulphonic acid. $Fe^{3+}+Ligand{\rightarrow}Complex$	Stable green colour.	Ferric

9. Ferrous

1.	Transfer 10 mg of the test substance into a test tube and add 2 ml water. Add 2 ml of dilute sulphuric acid and 1 ml of 0.1% w/v solution of 1,10 phenanthroline. $Fe^{2+}+Ligand\rightarrow Complex$ $Fe^{2+}+Ce^{4+}\rightarrow Fe^{3+}+Ce^{3+}$	Intense red colour. Discharged on addition of excess 0.1 M ceric ammonium sulphate.	Ferrous
2.	Transfer 10 mg of the test substance into a test tube and add 2 ml water. Add 1 ml of potassium ferri cyanide solution. $Fe^{2+}+[Fe(CN)_6]^{3-}\rightarrow Fe^{3+}+[Fe(CN)_6]^{4-}$ $4Fe^{3+}+3[Fe(CN)_6]^{4-}\rightarrow Fe_4[Fe(CN)_6]_3$ $Fe_4[Fe(CN)_6]_3+NaOH\rightarrow Fe(OH)_3+Na^++CN^-$	Dark blue precipitate. Insoluble in dilute hydrochloric acid. Decompose in sodium hydroxide solution.	Ferrous
3.	Transfer 10 mg of the test substance into a test tube and add 1 ml of potassium ferro cyanide solution. $Fe^{2+}+2K^++[Fe(CN)_6]^{4-}\rightarrow K_2Fe[Fe(CN)_6]$	White precipitate rapidly becomes blue and insoluble in dilute hydrochloric acid.	Ferrous

10. Lead

1.	Transfer 100 mg of the test substance into a test tube and add 1 ml of dilute acetic acid. Add 2 ml of potassium chromate solution. $PbSO_4+K_2CrO_4\rightarrow PbCrO_4$ $PbCrO_4+4NaOH\leftrightarrow[Pb(OH)_4]^{2-}+CrO_4^{2-}$	Yellow precipitate insoluble in 2 ml of 10 M sodium hydroxide	Lead
2.	Transfer 50 mg of the test substance into a test tube and add 1 ml of dilute acetic acid. Add 10 ml of water and 0.2 ml of 1 M potassium iodide. $Pb^{2+}+2I^-\rightarrow PbI_2$ $PbI_2+2I^-\leftrightarrow[PbI_4]^{2-}$	Yellow precipitate which on boiling and cooling form glistening yellow plates.	Lead

11. Magnesium

1.	Transfer 15 mg of the test substance into a test tube and add 2 ml of water. Add 1 ml of dilute ammonia solution. $MgSO_4+2NH_4OH\rightarrow$ $Mg(OH)_2 + (NH_4)_2SO_4$	White precipitate soluble in 1 ml 2 M ammonium chloride. White crystalline precipitate reappears on adding 1 ml of 0.25 M disodium hydrogen phosphate	Magnesium
2.	To 0.5 ml of a neutral or slightly acid solution of the substance, add 0.2 ml of a 0.1% w/v solution of titan yellow and 0.5 ml of 0.1M sodium hydroxide. $MgSO_4+2NaOH\rightarrow Mg(OH)_2$ Dye adsorbed on precipitate	Bright red turbidity gradually settles to a bright red precipitate.	Magnesium

12. Mercury

1.	Transfer 10 mg of the test substance into a test tube and add 0.5 ml water. Place the solution on a well scraped copper foil. $Cu+Hg^{2+}+Cu^{2+}+Hg$	Dark grey stain which shines on rubbing.	Mercury
2.	Transfer 10 mg of the test substance into a test tube and 0.5 ml water. Add potassium iodide solution. $Hg^{2+}+2I^-\rightarrow HgI_2$ $HgI_2+2I^-\rightarrow[HgI_4]^{2-}$	Red precipitate. soluble in excess reagent or yellow precipitate becoming green on standing.	Mercury
3.	Transfer 10 mg of the test substance into a test tube and add 0.5 ml water. Add 2 M sodium hydroxide until solution is alkaline. $Hg^{2+}+2OH^-\rightarrow HgO+H_2O$	Dense yellow precipitate.	Mercuric
4.	Transfer 10 mg of the test substance into a test tube and add 0.5 ml water. Add 6M hydrochloric acid. $HgNO_3+2HCl\rightarrow Hg_2Cl_2+HNO_3$ $Hg_2Cl_2+2NH_3\rightarrow Hg\downarrow+Hg(NH_2)Cl\downarrow+NH_4^++Cl^-$	White precipitate. Blackened by addition of dilute ammonia solution.	Mercurous

13. Potassium

1.	Transfer 50 mg of the test substance into a test tube and add 1 ml of water. Add 1 ml of dilute acetic acid and 1 ml of freshly prepared 10%w/v solution of sodium cobaltinitrite. $3K^{+}+[Co(NO_2)_6]^{3-}{\rightarrow}K_3[Co(NO_2)_6]\downarrow$	Yellow or orange – yellow precipitate	Potassium
2.	Transfer 100 mg of the test substance into a test tube and add 2 ml of water. Heat the solution with 1 ml of sodium carbonate solution. No precipitate is formed. Add 0.05 ml of sodium sulphide solution. No precipitate is formed. Cool in ice, add 2 ml of a 15 % w/v solution of tartaric acid. Allow to stand. $K^{+}+C_4H_6O_6{\leftrightarrow}KC_4H_5O_6\downarrow+H^{+}$ $K^{+}+C_4H_5O_6^{-}{\leftrightarrow}KC_4H_5O_6\downarrow$	White crystalline precipitate	Potassium
3.	Tranfer 100 mg of the test substance in a platinum crucible and ignite. Cool and dissolve in minimum quantity of water. Add 1 ml of platinic chloride solution in the presence of 1 ml of hydrochloric acid. $2K^{+}+[PtCl_6]^{2-}{\rightarrow}K_2[PtCl_6]\downarrow$	Yellow crystalline precipitate which on ignition leaves residue of potassium chloride on platinum.	Potassium

14. Silicates

Test	Observation	Inference
1. Transfer 200 mg of the test substance into a platinum crucible and add 10 mg of sodium fluoride and a few drops of sulphuric acid. Mix to form a slurry. Cover the crucible with a thin transparent plate of plastic under which a drop of water is suspended and warm gently. $Na_2SiO_3+4NaF+3H_2SO_4{\rightarrow}3Na_2SO_4+SiF_4+3H_2O$ $3SiF_4+2H_2O{\rightarrow}SiO_2\downarrow+2[SiF_6]^{2-}+4H^{+}$	A white ring is formed around the drop of water.	Silicates

15. Silver

1. Transfer 10 mg of the test substance into a test tube and add 10 ml water. Add 0.3 ml of dilute hydrochloric acid. $AgNO_3+HCl \rightarrow AgCl{\downarrow}+HNO_3$ $AgCl+KI \rightarrow AgI{\downarrow}+KCl$ $AgI+HNO_3 \rightarrow AgNO_3+HI$	A curdy white precipitate. Soluble in dilute ammonia. On adding potassium iodide solution forms yellow precipitate, soluble in nitric acid.	Silver

16. Sodium

1. Transfer 100 mg of the test substance into a test tube and add 2 ml of water. Add 2 ml of a 15% w/v solution of potassium carbonate and heat to boiling. No precipitate is produced. Add 4 ml of a freshly prepared potassium antimonate solution and heat to boiling. Allow to cool in ice and if necessary scratch the inside of the test-tube with a glass rod. (Sodium antimonite formation)	Dense white precipitate	Sodium
2. Transfer 100 mg of the test substance into a a test tube and 1 M acetic acid until solution is acidic. Add large excess of magnesium uranyl acetate solution. $Na^++Mg^{2+}+3UO_2^{2+}+9CH_3COO^- \rightarrow$ $NaMg(UO_2)_3(CH_3COO)_9{\downarrow}$ Sodium magnesium uranyl acetate	Yellow crystalline precipitate	Sodium

17. Zinc

1. Transfer 100 mg of the test substance into a test tube and add 5 ml of water. Add 0.2 ml of sodium hydroxide solution. $Zn^{2+}+2OH^- \leftrightarrow Zn(OH)_2\downarrow$ $Zn(OH)_2+2OH^- \leftrightarrow [Zn(OH)_4]^{2-}$ $Zn^{2+}+S^{2-} \rightarrow ZnS\downarrow$	White precipitate, dissolves in further addition of sodium hydroxide. White precipitate on addition of ammonium chloride and 0.1 ml of sodium sulphide solution.	Zinc
2. Transfer 100 mg of the test substance into a test tube and add 5 ml of water. Acidify with dilute sulphuric acid and add one drop of a 0.1% w/v solution of cupric sulphate and 2 ml of ammonium mercurithiocyanate solution. $CuSO_4+(NH_4)_2[Hg(SCN)_4]+ZnSO_4 \rightarrow$ $Zn[Hg(SCN)_4]+Cu[Hg(SCN)_4]$	Violet precipitate	Zinc
3. Transfer 100 mg of the test substance into a test tube and add 5 ml of water. Add 2 ml of potassium ferrocyanide solution. $3Zn^{2+}+2K^++2[Fe(CN)_6]^{4-} \rightarrow$ $K_2Zn_3[Fe(CN)_6]_2$	White precipitate in-soluble in dilute hydrochloric acid.	Zinc

Preparation of Reagents for Identification of Anions and Cations:

1. *0.05% w/v solution of quinalizarin in 1% w/v solution of sodium hydroxide:* A 0.05% w/v solution of quinalizarin in 1%w/v solution of sodium hydroxide.

2. *% w/v titan yellow solution:* A 0.1% w/v solution of titan yellow in water.

3. *M ceric ammonium sulphate solution:* Dissolve 6.3 g of ceric ammonium sulphate in 100 ml of water.

4. *M hydrochloric acid:* Solutions of any molarity x M may be prepared by diluting $85x$ ml of hydrochloric acid to 1000 ml with water.

5. *0.1 M iodine solution:* Solutions of x M may be prepared by dissolving $400x$ g of potassium iodide in the minimum amount of water, add $260x$ g of iodine, allow to dissolve and add sufficient water to produce 1000 ml.

6. *M silver nitrate solution:* Solutions of any molarity x M may be prepared by dissolving $170x$ g of silver nitrate in sufficient water to produce 1000 ml.

7. *M sodium hydroxide solution:* Solutions of x M may be prepared by dissolving $40x$ g of sodium hydroxide in sufficient water to produce 1000 ml.

8. *0.1% w/v 1,10 phenanthroline solution:* A 0.1% w/v solution of 1,10 phenanthroline in water.

9. *0.1% w/v mordant blue 3 solution:* 0.1% w/v solution of mordant blue 3 in water.

10. *M mercuric chloride solution:* Dissolve 54.30 g of mercuric chloride in 250 ml of dilute hydrochloric acid and make the volume to 1000 ml with water.

11. *0.2% w/v solution of 8-hydroxy-7-iodoquinoline-5-sulphonic acid:* Dissolve 0.2 g of 8-hydroxy-7-iodoquinoline-5-sulphonic acid in 100 ml of water.

12. *0.25 M disodium hydrogen phosphate solution:* Solutions of any molarity x M may be prepared by dissolving $358.15x$ g of disodium hydrogen phosphate in sufficient water to produce 1000 ml.

13. *% w/v ferrous sulphate solution:* 1.0% w/v solution of ferrous sulphate in freshly boiled and cooled water. The solution must be freshly prepared.

14. *M acetic acid solution:* Solutions of any molarity x M may be prepared by diluting $57x$ ml ($60x$ g) of glacial acetic acid to 1000 ml with water.

15. *M potassium iodide solution:* Dissolve 16. 6 g of potassium iodide in 100 ml of water.

16. *M sulphuric acid solution:* Solutions of x M may be prepared by carefully adding $54x$ ml of sulphuric acid to an equal volume of water and diluting to 1000 ml with water.

17. *10 % w/v sodium cobalti-nitrite solution:* A 10% w/v solution of sodium cobalti-nitrite in water.

18. *10 % w/v thiourea solution:* A 10 % w/v solution of thiourea in water.

19. *10 M ammonia solution:* Solutions of any molarity x M may be prepared by diluting $75x$ ml of strong ammonia solution to 1000 ml with water.

20. *10 M sodium hydroxide solution:* Solutions of any molarity x M may be prepared by dissolving $40x$ g of sodium hydroxide in sufficient water to produce 1000 ml.

21. *10% w/v sodium nitroprusside solution:* A 10% w/v solution of sodium nitroprusside in water.

22. *15% w/v potassium carbonate solution:* A 15% w/v solution of potassium carbonate in water.

23. *15% w/v tartaric acid solution:* A 15% w/v solution of tartaric acid in water.

24. *2% w/v ammonium oxalate solution:* A 2% w/v solution of ammonium oxalate in water.

25. *2% w/v resorcinol solution:* Shake 2 g of resorcinol with 100 ml of toluene until saturate and decant. Prepare immediately before use.

26. *M acetic acid solution:* Solutions of x M may be prepared by diluting $57x$ ml ($60x$ g) of glacial acetic acid to 1000 ml with water.

27. *M ammonium chloride solution:* Dissolve 106.98 g of ammonium chloride in sufficient water to produce 1000 ml.

28. *M hydrochloric acid:* Solutions of any molarity x M may be prepared by diluting $85x$ ml of hydrochloric acid to 1000 ml with water.

29. *M nitric acid solution:* Solutions of x M may be prepared by diluting $63x$ ml of nitric acid to 1000 ml with water.

30. *M sodium hydroxide solution:* A 20.0% w/v solution of sodium hydroxide in water.

31. *% sodium fluoride solution:* A 2.5% w/v solution of sodium fluoride in water.

32. *M acetic acid:* Solutions of any molarity x M may be prepared by diluting $57x$ ml ($60x$ g) of glacial acetic acid to 1000 ml with water.

33. *M hydrochloric acid solution:* Solutions of any molarity x M may be prepared by diluting $85x$ ml of hydrochloric acid to 1000 ml with water.

34. *Ammonium acetate solution:* Dissolve 150 g of ammonium acetate in 200 ml of water, add 3 ml of glacial acetic acid and dilute to 1000 ml with water. Use a freshly prepared solution.

35. *Ammonium carbonate solution:* Dissolve 5 g of ammonium carbonate in a mixture of 7.5 ml of dilute ammonia and 50 ml of water, dilute to 100 ml with water and filter, if necessary.

36. *Ammonium chloride solution:* A 10% w/v solution of ammonium chloride in water.

37. *Ammonium mercurithiocyanate solution:* Dissolve 30 g of ammonium thiocyanate and 27 g of mercuric chloride in sufficient water to produce 1000 ml.

38. *Ammonium thiocyanate solution:* A 10% w/v solution of ammonium thiocyanate in water.

39. *Barium chloride solution:* A 10.0% w/v solution of barium chloride in water.

40. Barium hydroxide solution: A 3.0% w/v solution of barium hydroxide in water.

41. *Bromine solution:* Dissolve 9.6 ml of bromine and 30 g of potassium bromide in sufficient water to produce 100 ml.

42. *Bromine water:* Freshly prepared saturated solution obtained by shaking occasionally during 24 hours 3 ml of bromine with 100 ml of water and allowing to separate. Store the solution over an excess of bromine, in light-resistant containers.

43. *Calcium chloride solution:* A 10.0% w/v solution of calcium chloride in water.

44. *Chlorine solution:* Saturated solution of chlorine in water. Chlorine is generated in Kipp's apparatus using bleaching powder lumps and hydrochloric acid.

45. *Dilute acetic acid solution:* Contains 6% w/w of glacial acetic acid. Dilute 57 ml of glacial acetic acid to 1000 ml with water.

46. *Dilute ammonia solution:* Contains approximately 10 % w/w of ammonia. Dilute 425 ml of strong ammonia solution to 1000 ml.

47. *Dilute hydrochloric acid solution:* Approximately 10 % w/w of hydrochloric acid in water.

48. *Dilute nitric acid solution:* Contains approximately 10 % w/w of nitric acid. Dilute 106 ml of nitric acid to 1000 ml with water.

49. *Dilute sodium hydroxide solution:* A 5.0% w/v solution of sodium hydroxide in water.

50. *Dilute sulphuric acid solution:* Contains approximately 10 % w/w of sulphuric acid. Dilute 57 ml of sulphuric acid to 1000 ml with water.

51. *Diphenyl carbazide solution:* Dissolve 0.2 g of 1,5-diphenyl carbazide in 10 ml of glacial acetic acid and dilute to 100 ml with ethanol.

52. *Ferric chloride solution:* A solution prepared from ferric chloride hexahydrate so as to contain about 15 % w/v of ferric chloride.

53. *Ferric chloride test solution:* 5.0% w/v solution of ferric chloride in water.

54. *Ferrous sulphate solution:* 2.0 % w/v solution of ferrous sulphate in freshly boiled and cooled water. The solution must be freshly prepared.

55. *Hydrogen peroxide (10 vol) solution:* Dilute hydrogen peroxide solution (20 vol) with an equal volume of water.

56. *Hypophosphorus reagent:* Dissolve, by heating gently, 10 g of sodium hypophosphite in 20 ml of water and dilute to 100 ml with hydrochloric acid. Allow to settle and decant or filter through glass wool.

57. *Iodine solution:* A 2.0 g of iodine and 3 g of potassium iodide in water to produce 100 ml.

58. *Lanthanum nitrate solution:* A 5% w/v solution of lanthanum nitrate in water.

59. *Lead acetate solution:* A 10.0% w/v solution of lead acetate in carbon-dioxide-free water.

60. *Magnesium sulphate solution:* A 5.0% w/v solution of magnesium sulphate in water.

61. *Magnesium uranyl acetate solution:* Heat on a water-bath 3.2 g of uranyl acetate, 10 g of magnesium acetate, 2 ml of glacial acetic acid and 30 ml of water. When solution is complete allow to cool, add 50 ml

of ethanol and dilute with water to 100 ml. Allow to stand for 24 hours and filter.

62. *Mercuric chloride solution:* A 5.0% w/v solution of mercuric chloride in water.

63. *Phenol solution:* A saturated solution of phenol in water.

64. *Platinic chloride solution:* A 5% w/v solution of chloroplatinic acid hexa hydrate in water.

65. *Potassium antimonite solution*: Boil 2 g of potassium antimonite with 95 ml of water until dissolved. Cool rapidly and add 50 ml of potassium hydroxide solution and 5 ml of 1 M sodium hydroxide. Allow to stand for 24 hours, filter and add sufficient water to produce 150 ml. Use freshly prepared solution.

66. *Potassium chromate solution:* A 5.0% w/v solution of potassium chromate in water.

67. *Potassium dichromate solution:* A 10.6% w/v solution of potassium dichromate in water.

68. *Potassium ferrocyanide solution:* A 5.0% w/v solution of potassium ferrocyanide in water.

69. *Potassium iodide solution:* A 16.6% w/v solution of potassium iodide in water.

70. *Potassium permanganate solution:* 3.0% w/v solution of potassium permanganate in water.

71. *Sodium hydroxide solution:* A 20.0% w/v solution of sodium hydroxide in water.

72. *Sodium sulphide solution:* A 10.0% w/v solution of sodium sulphide in water.

73. *Stannous chloride solution:* Dissolve 330 g of stannous chloride in 100 ml of hydrochloric acid and add sufficient water to produce 1000 ml.

74. *Thioacetamide reagent:* Add 1 ml of a mixture of 15 ml of 1 M sodium hydroxide, 5 ml of water and 20 ml of glycerin (85%) to 0.2 ml of thioacetamide solution, heat in a water-bath for 20 seconds, cool and use immediately.

6

Semi-Micro Analysis

Introduction to Semi-Micro Analysis of In-Organic Binary Mixtures

Qualitative analysis can be carried on various scales (i.e., quantity of test substance used for analysis). These are categorized as macro, semi-micro and microanalysis. In macro analysis about 0.1 to 0.5 g of test substance is used and volume taken for analysis is 20 ml. In semi-micro analysis about 0.01 to 0.05 g of test substance is used and volume taken for analysis is 10 ml (i.e., the quantities are reduced by factor 10-20). In micro-analysis the factor is of the order 100-200.

In binary mixture analysis, two anions and two cations present (unknown) are qualitatively analyzed and identified. Initially colour, odour provides some basic picture of nature of radicals that might be present in the unknown binary salt mixture, but not every time. Flame test is usually carried for preliminary identification of cations. In flame tests, the more volatile salts produced in the form of chlorides when exposed to non-luminous flame, the electrons (present in cations) gets excited from ground state to higher energy state (unstable state) by absorbing energy from heat. Once excited, the electrons try to procure the most stable form (i.e., the low energy state). During this process, the energy absorbed by the electrons is liberated out in the form of light energy (which is in visible range). No two cations have same characteristic flame colour. In case of binary mixtures, the colour of flame may not be good conclusion for identification of cations.

Tests like action on heating, action with dil. HCl and action with sulphuric acid gives clear picture of the presence of individual anions. Wet test i.e., sodium carbonate extract is prepared mainly to convert anions into the corresponding sodium salts which are easily soluble. In addition to this wet tests helps in identifying some of the anions (like sulphate) which cannot be identified in dry tests since acids like sulphuric acid is used. In some cases, wet tests help in identifying anions which are masked by presence of related other anions. One cannot use sodium carbonate extract for identification of carbonates/bi-carbonates since the extract itself is prepared using sodium carbonate and always gives positive to carbonates.

Once the two anions were identified, it is now to identify the two cations. Cations are separated from binary mixtures by selectively making them react with reagents. All the cations present in the periodic table were grouped into five categories based on their reaction with selective reagents. The main phenomenon applied is solubility and solubility product. Here, the less soluble product formed by reaction of cation and selective reagent is separated out first. The more soluble product is isolated and identified last.

Selective reagents like HCl, H_2S, NH_4Cl, NH_3, $(NH_4)_2CO_3$ are used in the group separation table. Hydrochloric acid and ammonia are used to selectively precipitate out the products of corresponding groups by common ion effect (a phenomenon of solubility and solubility product).

As we see, ammonia is used as a group reagent, one has to confirm presence of ammonium (NH_4^+) radical in the unknown binary mixture prior going to group separation.

Note:

One has to keep in mind that some of the anions (like borate, phosphate) interfere while performing group separation of cations. Hence, such interfering anions should be removed chemically and proceed further.

Systematic Layout of Group Separation of Cations:

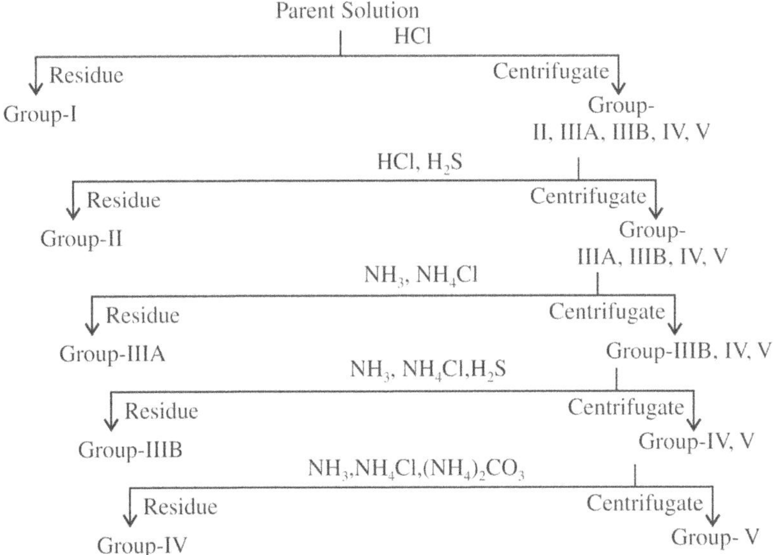

Cations: Ag^+ (Silver), Na^+ (Sodium), NH_4^+ (Ammonium), K^+ (Potassium), Ba^{2+} (Barium), Bi^{2+} (Bismuth), Ca^{2+} (Calcium), Cu^{2+} (Copper), Co^{2+} (Cobalt), Fe^{2+} (Ferrous), Hg^{2+} (Mercury), Pb^{2+} (Lead), Mg^{2+} (Magnesium), Mn^{2+} (Manganese), Ni^{2+} (Nickel), Sr^{2+} (Strontium), Zn^{2+} (Zinc), Al^{3+} (Aluminium), As^{3+} (Arsenic), Cr^{3+} (Chromium) and Fe^{3+} (Ferric).

Anions: Br^- (Bromide), Borates, Cl^- (Chloride), F^- (Fluoride), I^- (Iodide), CH_3COO^- (Acetate), NO^{2-} (Nitrite), NO^{3-} (Nitrate), CO_3^{2-} (Carbonate), $(COO)_2$ Oxalates, S^{2-} (Sulphide), SO_3^{2-} (Sulphite), SO_4^{2-} (Sulphate) and PO_4^{3-} (Phosphate), Tartarate $(C_4H_4O_6^{2-})$, $S_2O_3^-$ (thiosulphate).

A. Preliminary Tests

EXPERIMENT	OBSERVATION	INFERENCE
1. State:	i. Solid: Amorphous/ Crystalline/Hygroscopic	
	ii. Liquid	--------
2. Colour:	i. White (colour less)	May be Na^+, K^+, NH_4^+, Pb^{2+}, Al^{3+}, Zn^{2+}, Ba^{2+}, Ca^{2+}, Sr^{2+} or Mg^{2+} salt.
	ii. Blue or Bluish green colour	May be copper salts.
	iii. Pale green colour	May be ferrous salts.
	iv. Brown colour	May be ferric salt (hydrated form), bismuth, nickel, chromates or copper salt.
	v. Red or light pink color.	May be cobalt salt.
	vi. Colorless or slightly pinkish.	May be manganese salt.
	vii. Light green color.	May be nickel salt
	viii. Orange color.	May be chromates salt.
	ix. Yellow color	May be the salts of arsenic, chromates or ferric oxalate.
3. Appearance of the salt: Appearance of the given salt is noted.	i. Amorphous	May be carbonates, oxalates, phosphate, borates and fluorides.
	ii. Crystalline in nature.	Presence of chlorides, sulphates or nitrates.
4. Odour:	i. Smell of ammonia ($NH_3\uparrow$)	May be ammonium salts
	ii. Smell of vinegar (CH_3COOH)	May be acetate salts
	iii. Smell of rotten eggs (S^{2-})	May be sulphide salts

Contd

EXPERIMENT	OBSERVATION	INFERENCE
5. Solubility: Take a small quantity of the sample and check solubility in about 1ml a. Water b. Dil. HCl c. Conc. HCl d. Aqua-regia	 soluble/insoluble soluble/insoluble soluble/insoluble soluble/insoluble	 ------------ ------------ ------------ ------------
6. Flame test: Take a small quantity of test mixture on a watch glass, add 2-3 drops of conc. HCl. The paste is introduced into non-luminous flame with a glass rod. Observe the colour of the flame. (Note: Glass rod contains sodium) $BaSO_4 + HCl \rightarrow$ $BaCl_2 + H_2SO_4$	i. Golden yellow flame ii. Lilac flame iii. Brick red flame iv. Crimson flame v. Apple green flame	May be sodium(Na) May be potassium(K) May be calcium(Ca) May be strontium(Sr) May be barium(Ba)
7. Action on heating: Take a small quantity of the test mixture in a dry test-tube and heat.	i. Water droplets on the inner walls of the test tube. ii. Colour less gas, which turns limewater milky. $2NaHCO_3 \rightarrow Na_2CO_3 + H_2O + CO_2 \uparrow$ $CO_2 \uparrow + Ca(OH)_2 \rightarrow CaCO_3 \downarrow + H_2O$ iii. Cracking noise with reddish brown gas. $2NaNO_3 \rightarrow 2NaNO_2 + O_2 \uparrow$ $NH_4NO_3 \rightarrow N_2O \uparrow + 2H_2O$ $2AgNO_3 \rightarrow 2Ag + 2NO_2 \uparrow + O_2 \uparrow$ $2Pb(NO_3)_2 \rightarrow 2PbO + 4NO_2 \uparrow + O_2 \uparrow$	May be hydrated salts. May be carbonates, bi-carbonates May be halides, nitrates

Contd…

EXPERIMENT	OBSERVATION	INFERENCE
	iv. Water droplets on the inner walls of the test tube.	May be hydrated salts.
	v. Colour less gas, which turns limewater milky. $2NaHCO_3 \rightarrow Na_2CO_3 + H_2O + CO_2 \uparrow$ $CO_2 \uparrow + Ca(OH)_2 \rightarrow CaCO_3 \downarrow + H_2O$	May be carbonates, bi-carbonates
	vi. Cracking noise with reddish brown gas. $2NaNO_3 \rightarrow 2NaNO_2 + O_2 \uparrow$ $NH_4NO_3 \rightarrow N_2O \uparrow + 2H_2O$ $2AgNO_3 \rightarrow 2Ag + 2NO_2 \uparrow + O_2 \uparrow$ $2Pb(NO_3)_2 \rightarrow 2PbO + 4NO_2 \uparrow + O_2 \uparrow$	May be halides, nitrates
	vii. Colour less gas with rotten egg smell and turns lead acetate paper black. $Na_2S \rightarrow H_2S \uparrow$ $H_2S + Pb(CH_3COO)_2 \rightarrow$ $PbS \downarrow + 2CH_3COOH$	May be sulphides
	viii. Colour less gas with burning sulphur smell and turns potassium dichromate paper green. $SO_3^{2-} + 2H^+ \rightarrow SO_2 \uparrow + H_2O$ $3SO_3^{2-} + Cr_2O_7^{2-} + 8H^+ \rightarrow$ $2Cr^{3+} + 3SO_4^{2-} + 4H_2O$	May be sulphites, sulphates, thiosulphates.
	ix. Smell of vinegar. $CH_3COONH_4 \rightarrow CH_3COOH$	May be acetates.
	x. Smell of ammonia $[NH_4]_2CO_3 \rightarrow NH_3 \uparrow$	May be ammonia
	xi. Brown vapours, which turns starch paper yellow. $KBr \rightarrow Br_2$	May be bromides
	xii. Violet vapours which turns starch paper blue $KI \rightarrow I_2 \uparrow$	May be iodide.

B. Identification of Anions (Acidic Radicals) – Dry Tests

EXPERIMENT	OBSERVATION	INFERENCE
1. Action with dil. H₂SO₄: Take a small quantity of the test mixture in a dry test tube, add dil. H₂SO₄ drop wise. Heat gently.	i. Brisk effervescence, which turns limewater milky. $Na_2CO_3 + H_2SO_4 \rightarrow$ $Na_2SO_4 + H_2O + CO_2 \uparrow$ $2NaHCO_3 + H_2SO_4 \rightarrow$ $Na_2SO_4 + H_2O + CO_2$ $CO_2 + Ca(OH)_2 \rightarrow CaCO_3 \downarrow + H_2O$	May be carbonate, bi-carbonates
	ii. Colourless gas with rotten egg smell, which turns lead acetate paper black. $Na_2S + H_2SO_4 \rightarrow Na_2SO_4 + H_2S \uparrow$ $H_2S + Pb(CH_3COO)_2 \rightarrow$ $PbS + 2CH_3COOH$	May be sulphides.
	iii. Reddish-brown vapours, which turn starch iodide, paper bluish black. $2NaNO_2 + H_2SO_4 \rightarrow Na_2SO_4 + 2HNO_2 \uparrow$ $HNO_2 + 2HI \rightarrow I_2$ $I_2 + starch \rightarrow blue\ colour$	May be nitrites
	iv. Colour less gas with suffocating odour turning acidified potassium dichromate paper green. $SO_3^{2-} + 2H^+ \rightarrow SO_2 \uparrow + H_2O$ $3SO_3^{2-} + Cr_2O_7^{2-} + 8H^+ \rightarrow$ $2Cr^{3+} + 3SO_4^{2-} + 4H_2O$	May be sulphites.
	v. Colourless gas with smell of vinegar. $2CH_3COONa + H_2SO_4 \rightarrow$ $2CH_3COOH + Na_2SO_4$	May be acetates.

Contd…

EXPERIMENT	OBSERVATION	INFERENCE
2. Action with conc. H₂SO₄: Take a small quantity of the test mixture in a dry test tube, add conc. H₂SO₄ drop wise. Heat cautiously.	i. Colour less gas with pungent smell, which gives dense white fume on exposure to ammonia. (Use glass rod) $2NH_4Cl + H_2SO_4 \rightarrow$ $(NH_4)_2SO_4 + 2HCl \uparrow$ $HCl + NH_3 \rightarrow NH_4Cl \uparrow$	May be chlorides.
	ii. Reddish brown fumes which turns starch paper yellow. $2NaBr + H_2SO_4 \rightarrow Na_2SO_4 + 2HBr \uparrow$	May be bromides.
	iii. Reddish brown vapours which turn ferrous sulphate paper black. $4NO_3^- + 2H_2SO_4 \rightarrow$ $4NO_2 + O_2 + 2SO_4^{2-} + 2H_2O$	May be nitrates.
	iv. Violet vapours. $2KI + H_2SO_4 \rightarrow HI + HSO_4^-$ $3I^- + 2H_2SO_4 \rightarrow I_3^- + SO_4^{2-} +$ $2H_2O + SO_2$	May be iodides.
3. Action with MnO₂: Take a small quantity of the test mixture in a dry test tube, add equal quantity of MnO₂. Add drop wise 3-4 drops of conc. H₂SO₄. Heat gently.	i. Greenish yellow gas. Turns blue litmus red. $MnO(OH)_2 + 2H_2SO_4 + 2Cl^- \rightarrow$ $Mn^{2+} + Cl_2 + 2SO_4^{2-} + 3H_2O$	May be chlorides
	ii. Brown fumes. Turns starch iodide paper blue. Turns starch paper yellow. $2KBr + MnO_2 + 2H_2SO_4 \rightarrow$ $Br_2 + 2K^+ + Mn^{2+} + 2SO_4^{2-} + 2H_2O$	May be bromides.
	iii. Violet vapours. Turns starch paper blue. $3I^- + MnO_2 + 2H_2SO_4 \rightarrow$ $I_3^- + Mn^{2+} + 2SO_4^{2-} + 2H_2O$	May be iodides.

Contd…

EXPERIMENT	OBSERVATION	INFERENCE
4. Action with Cu and conc. H$_2$SO$_4$: Take a small quantity of the test mixture in a dry test tube, add 1 or 2 copper filings. Add conc. H$_2$SO$_4$ drop wise. Heat gently.	Brown fumes $2NO_3^- + 4H_2SO_4 + 3Cu \rightarrow$ $3Cu^{2+} + 2NO + 4SO_4^{2-} + 4H_2O$ $2NO + O_2 \rightarrow 2NO_2$	May be nitrates.
5. Test for phosphates: Take a small quantity of the test mixture in a dry test tube, add 5-6 drops of conc. HNO$_3$. Warm. Add excess solution of ammonium molybdate. Warm if necessary.	Canary yellow ppt. $HPO_4^{2-} + 3NH_4^{4+} + 12MoO_4^{2-} + 23H^+$ $\rightarrow (NH4)_3[P(Mo_3O_{10})_4]\downarrow + 12H_2O$	May be phosphates.
6. Test for borates: Take a small quantity of test mixture in a watch glass, add 4-5 drops of ethyl alcohol and 2-3 drops of conc. H$_2$SO$_4$. The paste is introduced into non-luminous flame with a glass rod.	Green-edged flame. $H_3BO_3 + 3C_2H_5OH \rightarrow B(OC_2H_5)_3 + 3H_2O$	May be borates.
7. Test for nitrites: Take a small quantity of test mixture in a test tube and dissolve in 0.5 ml of water. Add potassium permanganate solution (2 drops). Acidify with dil.HCl.	Potassium permanganate colour decolourises. $5NO_2^- + 2MnO_4^- + 6H^+ \rightarrow$ $5NO_3^- + 2Mn^{2+} + 3H_2O$	May be nitrites.

Contd…

EXPERIMENT	OBSERVATION	INFERENCE
8. Chromyl chloride test: (Test for chloride in presence of bromide) Take a small quantity of test mixture in a test tube and add equal quantity of potassium dichromate. Add conc.H_2SO_4 (5 drops) and warm gently.	Deep red vapours. $4Cl^- + Cr_2O_7^{2-} + 6H^+ \rightarrow 2CrO_2Cl_2 + 3H_2O$ $CrO_2Cl_2 + 4OH^- \rightarrow CrO_4^{2-} + 2Cl^- + 2H_2O$	May be chlorides.
9. Test for acetates: Take a small quantity of test mixture in a test tube and add $FeCl_3$ solution.	Deep red colouration or solution. $6CH_3COO^- + 3Fe^{3+} + 2H_2O \rightarrow$ $[Fe_3(OH)_2(CH_3COO)_6]^+ + 2H^+$ $[Fe_3(OH)_2(CH_3COO)_6]^+ + 4H_2O \rightarrow$ $3Fe(OH)_2CH_3COO\downarrow + 3CH_3COOH + H^+$	May be acetates.

C. Wet Tests

EXPERIMENT	OBSERVATION	INFERENCE
Preparation of Na$_2$CO$_3$ extract: Take about 0.1 g of test mixture in a test tube, add 0.3 g of sodium carbonate and 10ml water, boil the contents for 5 mins, cool and filter. The filterate is known as sodium carbonate extract.	$BaSO_4$(in-soluble) + $Na_2CO_3 \rightarrow$ Na_2SO_4 (soluble) + $BaCO_3$	-------------
1. Test for halides: To 0.5ml of extract, add dil. HNO$_3$ until acidic. Add 1-2 drops of silver nitrate solution.	i. White ppt. Soluble in dil. NH$_3$. Soluble in dil. HNO$_3$ $NaCl + AgNO_3 \rightarrow AgCl\downarrow + NaNO_3$ $AgCl + 2NH_3 \rightarrow [Ag(NH_3)_2]^+ + Cl^-$ $AgCl + HNO_3 \rightarrow AgNO_3 + HNO_3$ ii. Pale yellow ppt. Sparingly soluble in dil.NH$_3$. Insoluble in dil.HNO$_3$ $NaBr + AgNO_3 \rightarrow AgBr\downarrow + NaNO_3$ iii. Yellow ppt. Insoluble in dil. NH$_3$. Insoluble in dil. HNO$_3$ $NaI + AgNO_3 \rightarrow AgI\downarrow + NaNO_3$ iv. Yellow ppt. Soluble in dil. HNO$_3$ $HPO_4^{2-} + 3Ag^+ \rightarrow Ag_3PO_4 + H^+$ $Ag_3PO_4 + 2H^+ \rightarrow H_2PO_4^- + 3Ag^+$ $Ag_3PO_4 + 6NH_3 \rightarrow$ $3[Ag(NH_3)_2]^+ + PO_4^{3-}$	Chlorides confirmed Bromides confirmed Iodides confirmed Phosphate confirmed

Contd...

2. Brown-ring test: Take 0.5 ml of extract and add equal amount ferrous sulphate solution. Add drop wise conc. H_2SO_4 from side of test tube.	Brown-ring at junction of two layers $2NO_3^- + 4H_2SO_4 + 6Fe^{2+}$ $\rightarrow 6Fe^{3+} + 2NO + 4SO_4^{2-} + 4H_2O$ $Fe^{2+} + NO \rightarrow [Fe(NO)]^{2+}$	Nitrates confirmed.
3. Test for sulphates: Take 0.5 ml of extract and add dil. HCl until acidic. Add 1-2 drops of barium chloride solution.	White ppt. Insoluble in dil. HCl. Insoluble in dil. HNO_3. $SO_4^{2-} + BaCl_2 \rightarrow BaSO_4 \downarrow + 2Cl^-$	Sulphate confirmed.
4. Test for bromide in presence of iodide : (Test for bromide and iodide in presence of each other and of chloride) Take 0.5 ml of extract, acidify with dil. HCl, add 1-2 drops of chlorine water and 1 ml of chloroform. Shake. Observe chloroform layer. Add further dropwise chlorine water. (Note: Chloride do not interfere the test)	i. Violet colour in the chloroform layer. $3I^- + Cl_2 \rightarrow I_3^- + 2Cl^-$ ii. Violet colour disappeared and reddish brown colour in the chloroform layer. $I_3^- + 8Cl_2 + 9H_2O \rightarrow$ $3IO_3^- + 16Cl^- + 18H^+$ $2Br^- + Cl_2 \rightarrow Br_2 + 2Cl^-$ $Br_2 + Cl_2 \leftrightarrow 2BrCl$	Iodide confirmed. Bromide confirmed.
5. Test for nitrate in presence of bromide and/or iodide: Take 0.5 ml of extract, add 0.5 ml dil. NaOH. Boil until smell of ammonia ceases. Add Al powder (or wire). Warm gently.	Ammonia smell. Turns red litmus blue. $3NO3^- + 8Al + 5OH^- + 18H_2O \rightarrow$ $NH_3 + 4[Zn(OH)_4]^{2-}$	Nitrate confirmed.

Contd...

6. Test for chloride in presence of bromide and/or iodide: Take 0.5 ml of extract, add 2 M acetic acid until solution is acidic. Add lead dioxide and boil the mixture until bromine and iodine are no longer evolved. Filter. To the filterate add dil. HNO_3 and 1-2 drops of $AgNO_3$.	White ppt. Soluble in dil. NH_3 Insoluble in dil. HNO_3 $2Br^-+PbO_2+4CH_3COOH\rightarrow$ $Br_2+Pb^{2+}+4CH_3COO^-+2H_2O$ $3I^-+PbO_2+4CH_3COOH\rightarrow$ $I_3^-+Pb^{2+}+4CH_3COO^-+2H_2O$ $Cl^-+AgNO_3\rightarrow AgCl+NO_3^-$	Chloride confirmed
7. Test for chloride in presence of iodide: Take 0.5 ml of extract and acidify with dil. HNO_3. Add 3-4 drops of $AgNO_3$ solution (add excess if necessary). Filter. Reject the filterate. Wash the precipitate with dil. NH_3 and filter again. Add dil. HNO_3 to the filterate.	White ppt. $Cl^-+AgNO_3\rightarrow AgCl+NO_3^-$ $I^-+AgNO_3\rightarrow AgI+NO_3^-$ $AgCl+AgI+2NH_3\rightarrow$ $[Ag(NH_3)_2]^+(soluble)+Cl^- +$ $AgI(insoluble\ in\ ammonia)$	Chloride confirmed
8. Test for nitrate in presence of nitrite: Take 0.5ml of extract and add 50mg of solid sulphamic acid. Add equal volume of $FeSO_4$ solution. Add drop wise conc. H_2SO_4 from side of test tube.	Brown-ring at junction of two layers $HO.SO_2.NH_2+HNO_2\rightarrow$ $N_2\uparrow+2H^++SO_4^{2-}+H_2O$ $2NO_3^-+4H_2SO_4+6Fe^{2+}\rightarrow$ $6Fe^{3+}+2NO\uparrow+4SO_4^{2-}+4H_2O$ $Fe^{2+}+NO\uparrow\rightarrow[Fe(NO)]^{2+}$	Nitrates confirmed.

Contd…

9. Test for acetates: Take 0.5ml of extract and acidify with conc. H_2SO_4. Add 2 to 4 drops of amyl alcohol (or ethyl alcohol) and heat. (Make sure the solution is acidic)	Fruity odour $RCOOH+R_1OH \rightarrow RCOOR+H_2O$	Acetates confirmed.

D. Identification of Cations (Basic Radicals)

1. Test for Ammonium (NH_4^+)

EXPERIMENT	OBSERVAION	INFERENCE
i. Take a small quantity of test mixture in a test tube and add 0.5 ml dil. NaOH and warm.	Smell of Ammonia. Vapours turn red litmus paper blue. Dense white fumes when a glass rod moistened with conc. HCl is held in the vapour. $(NH_4)_2SO_4+2NaOH \rightarrow$ $Na_2SO_4+2NH_3\uparrow+2H_2O$ $NH_3+HCl \rightarrow NH_4Cl$	Ammonium salts
ii. Test with Nessler's reagent: Take a small quantity of test mixture in a test tube and dissolve in 0.5 ml of water. Add 2-3 drops of Nessler's reagent.	Reddish brown ppt. $NH_4^+ +2[HgI_4]^{2-}+4OH^- \rightarrow$ $HgO.Hg(NH_2)I\downarrow+7I^-+3H_2O$ (Mercury(II) amido-iodine)	Ammonium salts.

Systematic Separation of Cations (Basic Radicals)

Preparation of Sample Solution (Parent Solution)

1. *Solution in water:* Take a small quantity of test mixture in test tube and add about $1/3^{rd}$ test-tube of water, shake well and boil. If the mixture dissolves completely, the components of mixture are water-soluble. In such case the aqueous solution of mixture is used as such for analysis (i.e. proceeding for group separation)

2. *Solution in dil. HCl :* If the mixture is not completely soluble in water, take small quantity of mixture in test-tube and add about 10 ml of dil.HCl, boil the mixture. If the mixture dissolves completely, then use this solution for analysis from Group-II on-wards. If gas like CO_2 or H_2S etc., is evolved, boil the solution to remove the gas completely.

3. *Solution in Conc. HCl :* Take a small quantity of mixture in test-tube and add 5 ml conc. HCl. Boil the mixture carefully. If gas is evolved, remove it by boiling. Dilute this solution carefully after cooling, with water and use for further analysis.

4. *Solution in Aqua regia :* If the given mixture is insoluble in acids, solution in aqua regia is carried out. Take a small quantity of mixture in test-tube, add 2-3 ml aqua regia. Boil the contents, cool and then carefully dilute with water. The solution is used for further analysis.

Group Separation Table

Parent solution: Add a few drops of dil.HCl (cold). If a precipitate (residue) forms, continue adding dil.HCl until no further precipitation takes place. Centrifuge.

White ppt

Group I

Pb Cl$_2$

Ag Cl

Hg$_2$ Cl$_2$

Centrifugate: Add 1ml of 3% v/v H$_2$O$_2$ solution. Add dil. HCl until solution is acidic. Heat to boiling. Pass H$_2$S gas until solution becomes saturated. Centrifuge. (repeat until no further precipitation takes place)

Coloured ppt

Group II

HgS, PbS,

Bi$_2$S$_3$, CuS

CdS, As$_2$S$_3$

Sb$_2$S$_3$, Sb$_2$S$_5$

SnS, SnS$_2$

Centrifugate: Boil in a porcelain dish (or test-tube) and ensure all H$_2$S has been removed (test with lead acetate paper). Add 3-4 drops of dil.HNO$_3$. Heat gently. Add dil. NH$_4$Cl and dil. NH$_3$ solution until solution is alkaline. Centrifuge.

Coloured ppt

Group III A

Fe(OH)$_3$

Cr(OH)$_3$

Al(OH)$_3$

Centrifugate: Add dil.NH$_3$ solution until solution is alkaline. Heat. Pass H$_2$S gas until saturation. Centrifuge.

Coloured ppt

Group III B

CoS, NiS,

MnS, ZnS

Centrifugate: Boil in a porcelain dish (or in a test-tube) and ensure all H$_2$S has been removed. Add NH$_4$Cl and dil. NH$_3$ solution (until alkaline) and (NH$_4$)$_2$CO$_3$ solution in excess.

White ppt.

Group IV

BaCO$_3$

SrCO$_3$

CaCO$_3$

Centrifugate: Transfer into a china-dish and evaporate to dryness. Add 1ml of dil.HNO$_3$, evaporate to dry-ness.

White ppt.

Group V

NaNO$_3$, KNO$_3$, Mg(NO$_3$)$_2$, NH$_4$NO$_3$

Separation and Identification of Group-I Cations (Silver Group)

Residue(ppt): Contains $PbCl_2$, $AgCl$ and Hg_2Cl_2. Wash with dil.HCl, then with 1ml of cold water (2 to 3 times) and reject the washings. Boil the residue with 2ml water. Centrifuge when hot.

Residue: May contain Hg_2Cl_2 and AgCl. Wash the residue several times with hot water until the washings give no ppt with K_2CrO_4 solution. This ensures complete removal of the Pb.

Pour 2-3 ml of dil. NH_3 solution over the precipitate and centrifuge

---

Residue:

Black

$Hg(NH_2)Cl + Hg$

Hg_2^{2+} present

Centrifugate:
May contain $[Ag(NH_3)_2]^+$

Divide into 2 parts:

1. To one part add dil.HNO_3 until solution is acidic.

    White ppt.
    AgCl

2. To second part add KI solution dropwise.

    Yellow ppt.
    Ag present

Centrifugate: May contain $PbCl_2$. Cool the solution and divide into 3 parts.

1. To one part add potassium chromate solution, dropwise.

    Yellow ppt,
    insoluble in dil.AcOH
    $PbCrO_4$

2. To second part add potassium iodide solution, drop wise.

    Yellow ppt.
    Soluble on boiling and
    on cooling gives brilliant yellow crystals.
    PbI_2

3. To third part add dil. H_2SO_4 until solution is acidic.
    White ppt $PbSO_4 \downarrow$
    Soluble in ammonium acetate solution.
    $(CH_3COO)_2Pb$
    Pb present

Separation and Identification of Group-II Cations

Residue: Contains HgS, PbS, Bi₂S₃, CuS, CdS, As₂S₃, Sb₂S₃, Sb₂S₅, SnS, SnS₂. Wash with little of NH₄Cl solution, discard washings. Add about 5 ml of yellow ammonium poly sulphide solution, heat to 50-60 C with constant stirring. Centrifuge.

Residue: Group-II A present.
Contains HgS, PbS, Bi₂S₃, CuS and CdS. Wash with dil. ammonium sulphide solution. Wash with 2% w/v NH₄NO₃ solution. Discard all washings. Add 4 ml of dil. HNO₃. Boil gently for 2-3 minutes. Centrifuge.

Centrifugate: Group-IIB

Residue:
Black.

HgS.

Dissolve the residue with a mixture of 0.5 ml sodium hypochlorite solution and 0.5 ml dil. HCl. Boil off excess chlorine. Add SnCl₂ solution dropwise.

White ppt turning grey or black.

Hg²⁺ present

Centrifugate: Contains nitrates of Pb, Bi, Cu and Cd. Test a small portion for Pb by adding dil. H₂SO₄ and alcohol. White ppt indicates Pb present. If Pb present, add dil. H₂SO₄ to the remaining centrifugate.

Residue:
White
PbSO₄
Add ammonium acetate solution. Centrifuge. To the centrifugate add dil. AcOH. Add potassium chromate solution dropwise.

Yellow ppt.

PbCrO₄

Pb present.

Centrifugate: Contains nitrates and sulphates of Bi, Cu and Cd. Add strong NH₃, until solution is alkaline (highly alkaline). Centrifuge.

Residue:

White
Bi(OH)₃

Dissolve in dil. HCl and add sodium tetrahyroxo-stannate(II) dropwise.

Black ppt.

Bi present

Centrifugate:
Contains [Cu(NH₃)₄]²⁺ and/or [Cd(NH₃)₄]²⁺
Deep blue colour.
Cu present.

1. To one part add dil. AcOH and potassium ferro cyanide solution. Reddish brown ppt. Cu present.

2. To second part add KCN solution drop-wise until colour is discharged. Add further in excess. Pass H₂S gas.
    Yellow ppt
    CdS
    Cd present

Centrifugate: Group IIB

Add dil.HCl with constant stirring until slightly acidic. Warm and shake. A fine white or yellow precipitate is sulphur only. A yellow or orange flocculant precipitate indicates As, Sb and Sn present. Centrifuge and wash the precipitate (which may contain As_2S_5, As_2S_3, Sb_2S_5 and S) with a little H_2S water, reject the washings.

To the residue add 3 ml of conc. HCl and boil gently for 1 minute (to reprecipitate small amounts of arsenic that may have dissolved). Centrifuge.

Residue: Contains As_2S_5, As_2S_3 and S (yellow).	**Centrifugate:**
1. Dissolve in 2 ml of warm dil.NH_3 solution. Add 1ml of 3% v/v H_2O_2 solution and warm for few minutes (oxidizes Arsenite to Arsenate). Add magnesium nitrate reagent dropwise. Stir and allow to stand.	1. To one part add dil.NH_3 solution and make alkaline. Add small quantity of (20 mg) of oxalic acid, boil. Centrifuge. Pass H_2S gas into centrifugate.
White crystalline ppt.	Orange ppt.
$Mg(NH_4)AsO_4.6H_2O$	Sb_2S_3
As present.	Sb present
2. Take the above-obtained residue, add 6-7 drops dil. AcOH. Add silver nitrate solution drop-wise.	2. To second part add dil.NH_3 until solution is partially neutral. Add small quantity of magnesium powder. Warm gently. Centrifuge. Add mercuric chloride solution.
Brownish red ppt.	White ppt or grey ppt
Ag_3AsO_4	Hg_2Cl_2 or Hg
	Sn present

Removal of borates:

(a) If borate and fluoride are present, evaporate the residue repeatedly with 5-10 ml conc. HCl.

(b) If borate is present and fluoride is absent, treat with 1 ml methanol and 2 ml conc. HCl and evaporate on a water bath.

Separation and Identification of Group-IIIA

Residue: Contains $Fe(OH)_3$, $Cr(OH)_3$, $Al(OH)_3$ and a little of $MnO(OH)_2$. Wash with a little hot NH_4Cl solution.

To the residue add 2 ml of water, add 1.5 ml of 10% w/v NaOH solution and 1.5 ml 3% v/v H_2O_2 solution. Boil gently until the evolution of O_2 ceases (2-3) minutes. Centrifuge.

Residue: Contains $Fe(OH)_3$, $MnO(OH)_2$. Wash with a little hot water.	**Centrifugate:** Contains CrO_4^{2-} (yellow) and $[Al(OH)_4]^{-}$ (colour less)
1. To small portion of ppt in 1ml of dil. HNO_3, add 3-4 drops of 3% v/v H_2O_2 solution. Boil, cool thoroughly and add 50 mg of sodium bismuthate. Shake and allow the solid to settle. Violet solution MnO_4^{-} Mn present	If the solution is colour less, Cr is absent. If solution is yellow, Cr is present. Divide into 3 parts
	1. To one part add dil.AcOH and lead acetate solution. Yellow ppt ($PbCrO_4$) Cr present
2. To another portion of the ppt, add dil. HCl. Add 1 or 2 drops of NH_4SCN solution. Deep red coloration Fe present	2. To second part add dil.HNO_3 until acidic. Cool. Add 1ml amyl alcohol and 4 drops of H_2O_2 solution. Shake well and allow the two layers to separate. Blue upper layer Cr present.
3. To another portion of the ppt, add dil. HCl. Add 1 or 2 drops of potassium ferro cyanide solution. Blue ppt. Fe present.	
	3. To third part add dil.HCl until acidic. Add dil. NH_3 solution until just alkaline. Heat to boiling. Centrifuge. White gelatinous ppt. $Al(OH)_3$ Al present
4. Test for Fe^{3+} and Fe^{2+}: (a) Take a small quantity of test mixture and dissolve in 1ml water. Add 1 or 2 drops of potassium ferro cyanide solution. Deep blue ppt. $Fe_4[Fe(CN)_6]_3$ Fe^{3+} present	
(b) Take small quantity of test mixture add 1 ml of water and dissolve. Add ammonium thiocyanate solution dropwise. No colour Fe^{2+} present Deep red colour, $Fe(SCN)_3$, Fe^{3+} present	4. Take a small portion of the above ppt. and add 1 ml of dil.HCl. To the clear solution add 1 ml ammonium acetate solution and 0.5 ml of aluminon reagent. Stir. Add ammonium carbonate solution until basic. Red ppt. Al present.

Separation and Identification of Group-IIIB Cations

Residue: Contains CoS, NiS, MnS and ZnS. Wash the residue thoroughly with equal volumes of NH_4Cl and $(NH_4)_2S$ solution and discard washings after centrifuge. To the residue add 3 ml water and 3 ml dil.HCl. Stir. Allow to stand for 2-3 minutes. Centrifuge.

Residue: Contains CoS and NiS. To the ppt. in a test tube add 1 ml of NaOCl solution and 0.5 ml dil.HCl, boil until Cl_2 expelled out. Cool and dilute to 4 ml.

Divide the solution into two equal parts.

1. To one part add 1ml amyl alcohol, 100 mg of solid NH_4SCN and shake well.

Blue colour
in amyl alcohol layer.

Co present.

2. To second part add NH_4Cl solution. Add dil. NH_3 solution dropwise until the solution is alkaline. Add excess of di-methyl glyoxime reagent.

Ni present

Centrifugate: Contains Mn^{2+} and Zn^{2+} and possibly traces of Co^{2+} and Ni^{2+}. Boil until H_2S removed (test fumes with lead acetate paper). Cool, add excess dil. NaOH solution. Add 1ml of 3% v/v H_2O_2 solution. Boil. Centrifuge.

Residue:
Contains largely $MnO(OH)_2$, traces of $Ni(OH)_2$ and $Co(OH)_2$.

1. To part of the residue add dil. HNO_3 until solution is obtained. Add 5 drops of H_2O_2 solution. Boil thoroughly, cool. Add 50 mg of $NaBiO_3$. Stir and allow to settle.

Purple solution.
MnO_4^-
Mn present.

Centrifugate:
Contains $[Zn(OH)_4]^{2-}$
Divide into 2 parts.

1 To one part add dil. AcOH and pass H_2S gas.
White ppt
ZnS
Zn present.

2. To second part add dil. H_2SO_4 and acidify. Add 0.5 ml cobalt acetate solution and 0.5 ml of ammonium tetra thiocyanato mercurate (II) reagent. Stir.
Pale blue ppt.
Zn present.

Separation and Identification of Group IV Cations

Residue: Contains $BaCO_3$, $SrCO_3$ and $CaCO_3$. Wash with hot water and reject washings. To the residue add 5 ml of dil. AcOH and dissolve. Take a small part (0.5 ml) of the solution, add potassium chromate solution dropwise. Boil. Yellow ppt indicates, barium.

If Barium present: Heat the remainder of the solution to boiling and add slight excess of potassium chromate solution (i.e., until solution assumes yellow colour). Centrifuge. Wash the residue (ppt) with hot water.

If Barium absent: Discard the portion used in testing for barium, and employ the remainder of solution, after boiling for 1 min to expel CO_2, to test for strontium and calcium.

| **Residue:**
Yellow . Contains $BaCrO_4$.
Wash the residue with hot water.

1. Take a small portion of the residue and dissolve in conc. HCl. Evaporate in a china-dish until a paste is formed. Introduce the paste in the non-luminous flame of Bunsen burner.

Apple green or yellowish green flame.

Ba present.

2. Flame Test: Perform with direct test mixture.

Apple green flame

Ba present. | **Centrifugate:** Sr and Ca.
If barium present: Add dil. NH_3 solution until alkaline and then add $(NH_4)_2CO_3$ solution in excess. White ppt indicates $SrCO_3$ and /or $CaCO_3$. Wash the residue with hot water and dissolve in 3 ml of dil. AcOH. Boil to remove excess CO_2.
or
If barium absent: Boil the solution to remove CO_2.

To either of the solutions add equal vol. of saturated $(NH_4)_2SO_4$ solution, add 0.2 g sodium thiosulphate. Heat in a water bath for 5 min and allow to stand for 5 min. (Add triethanolamine if necessary) |

| | **Residue:**
Contains $SrSO_4$.
Wash the residue with water.
1. Transfer the residue into a watch glass and add conc. HCl. Introduce paste in non luminous flame.

Crimson flame
Sr present. | **Centrifugate:** Contains Ca.
1. To a part of solution add dil. AcOH and ammonium oxalate solution dropwise. Warm on a water bath.

White ppt.
CaC_2O_4
Ca present.

2. Flame test: Perform with direct test mixture.

Brick red flame
Ca present. |

Separation and Identification of Group-V Cations

Residue: Dissolve the residue obtained in about 5 ml water. Divide into 3 parts. To one portion add 2% w/v 8-hydroxy-quinoline solution and dil. NH_3 until solution is highly alkaline. (If Mg present, do for the whole solution).

(If Mg present or absent use the other two portions for testing K, Na respectively)

Residue:	**Centrifugate:** Contains K, Na.
Contains Mg.	Divide each part into two parts.
Dissolve the residue in 0.5 ml of dil. HCl and add 2-3 ml water.	
	1. To one part add dropwise uranyl magnesium acetate reagent. Shake and allow to stand for a few minutes
Divide the solution into two parts	
1. To one part add 2% 8-hydroxy quinoline solution in 2M AcOH with 3 ml of dil.NH_3 solution (if necessary warm to dissolve any ppt formed). Add a little of NH_4Cl solution. Add ammonical oxine reagent. Heat to boiling until smell of ammonia disappears.	Yellow crystalline ppt. Na present.
	2. Flame test: Perform with direct test mixture.
Pale yellow ppt. Mg'oxinate' Mg present.	Golden yellow flame Na present.
	3. To one part add dropwise (2-3drops) sodium hexanitrito cobaltate. Add 4-5 drops of dil.AcOH. Stir. Allow to stand for 1-2 min.
2. To one part add 2 drops of the Magneson reagent. Add few drops of dil.NaOH until solution is alkaline.	Yellow ppt $K_3[Co(NO_2)_6]$ K present
	4. Flame test: Perform with direct test mixture.
Blue ppt.	Lilac flame
Mg confirms.	K present.

Preparation of Reagents for Semi-Micro Analysis

1. *10% sodium hydroxide solution:* A 10 %w/v solution of sodium hydroxide in water.

2. *2 M acetic acid solution:* Solution of xM may be prepared by diluting $57x$ ml ($60x$ g) of glacial acetic acid to 1000 ml water.

3. *2% 8-hydroxy quinoline solution in 2 M acetic acid: A* 2% w/v solution of 8-hydroxy quinoline in 2 M acetic acid.

4. *2% Ammonium nitrate solution:* A 2% w/v solution of ammonium nitrate in water.

5. *Aluminon reagent:* Dissolve 0.1 g of aluminon (tri-ammonium arurine-tricarboxylate) in 100 ml water.

6. *Ammonical oxime reagent- oxine reagent :* A 2% w/v 8-hydroxy quinoline in acetic acid.

7. *Ammonium acetate solution:* A 5% w/v solution of ammonium acetate in water.

8. *Ammonium carbonate solution*: A 5% w/v solution of ammonium carbonate in water.

9. *Ammonium molybdate solution:* Dissolve 4.4 g ammonium molybdate in a mixture of 6 ml of concentrated ammonia and 4 ml of water. Add 12 g of ammonium nitrate and after complete dissolution dilute the solution to 100 ml.

10. *Ammonium oxalate solution:* A 5% w/v solution of ammonium oxalate in water.

11. *Ammonium poly sulphide solution:* To 1 litre 1 M solution of ammonium sulphide add 32 g sulphur, and heat gently until the latter dissolves completely and a yellow solution is formed.

12. *Ammonium tetra thiocyanato mercurate reagent:* Dissolve 9 g of ammonium thiocyanate and 8 g of mercury(II) chloride, in water and dilute to 100ml with water.

13. *Ammonium thiocyanate solution:* A 5% w/v solution of ammonium thiocyanate in water.

14. *Aqua-regia:* To 3 volumes of concentrated hydrochloric acid add 1 volume of concentrated nitric acid. Mix and use immediately. Prepare fresh solution when necessary.

15. *Barium chloride solution:* A 5% w/v solution of barium chloride in water.

16. *Chlorine gas:* The gas is generated in Kipp's apparatus using calcium hypochlorite (bleaching powder) and 5 M hydrochloric acid. The bleaching powder is mixed with gypsum powder, making the mixture wet, to produce lumps of the reagent. After drying these lumps are used in Kipp's apparatus.

17. *Chlorine water:* Saturated solution of chlorine gas in water.

18. *Dilute acetic acid:* A 5% v/v solution of glacial acetic acid in water.

19. *Dilute ammonia solution:* A 5% v/v solution of strong ammonia solution in water.

20. *Dilute ammonium chloride solution:* A 5% w/v solution of ammonium chloride in water.

21. *Dilute ammonium sulphide solution:* A 5% w/v solution of ammonium sulphide in water.

22. *Dilute hydrochloric acid:* A 5% v/v solution of concentrated hydrochloric acid in water.

23. *Dilute nitric acid:* A 5%v/v solution of concentrated nitric acid in water.

24. *Dilute sodium hydroxide:* A 5% w/v solution of sodium hydroxide in water.

25. *Dilute sulphuric acid:* A 5% v/v solution of concentrated sulphuric acid in water.

26. *Dimethyl glyoxime reagent:* A 1% w/v solution of dimethyl glyoxime in ethanol (95%).

27. *Ferrous sulphate paper:* In a 5% w/v ferrous sulphate in 5% v/v solution of sulphuric acid in water, dip filter paper.

28. *Ferrous sulphate solution:* A 5% w/v solution of ferrous sulphate in 5% v/v solution of sulphuric acid in water.

29. *Hydrogen sulphide gas:* The gas is generated in Kipp's apparatus using ferrous sulphide sticks and 1:1 volumes of concentrated hydrochloric acid and water.

30. *Lead acetate paper:* A filter paper dipped in 5% w/v solution of lead acetate.

31. *Lead acetate solution:* A 5% w/v solution of lead acetate in 1-5% v/v of glacial acetic acid in water.

32. *Lime water:* A 5% w/v solution of calcium hydroxide in carbon di-oxide free water and filter the un-dissolved.   The solution has to be prepared quickly under carbon di-oxide free atmosphere.

33. *Magnesium nitrate solution:* A 5% w/v solution of magnesium nitrate in water.

34. *Magneson reagent:* A 0.5% w/v 4-(4-nitro phenyl azo)-resorcinol-(Magneson I) reagent in 2% w/v sodium hydroxide solution.

35. *Nessler's reagent:* Dissolve 10 g of potassium iodide in 10 ml of water (solution a). Dissolve 6 g of mercury (II) chloride in 100 ml water (solution b). Dissolve 45 g potassium hydroxide in water and dilute to 80 ml (solution c). Add solution b to solution a dropwise until a slight permanent precipitate is formed, then add solution c, mix and dilute with water to 200 ml. Allow to stand overnight and decant the clear solution.

36. *Potassium chromate solution:* A 5% w/v solution of potassium chromate in water.

37. *Potassium cyanide solution:* POISON. A 1% w/v solution of potassium cyanide in water. Prepare minimum volumes as per requirement and decompose excess left over reagent in excess potassium permanganate solution in water. If permanganate solution is in brown colour on decomposition indicates insufficient potassium permanganate. On decomposition the colour of decomposed solution should be always purple in colour.

38. *Potassium dichromate paper:* A filter paper dipped in 5% w/v solution of potassium dichromate solution.

39. *Potassium dichromate solution:* A 5% w/v solution of potassium dichromate in water.

40. *Potassium ferrocyanide solution:* A 5% w/v solution of potassium ferro cyanide in water.

41. *Potassium iodide solution:* A 5% w/v solution of potassium iodide in water.

42. *Saturated ammonium sulphate solution:* Dissolve ammonium sulphate in 100 ml water until no further ammonium sulphate dissolves in the solution. Filter the solution and use. Prepare fresh solution if necessary.

43. *Silver nitrate solution:* A 1% w/v solution of silver nitrate in halide free water.

44. *Sodium hexanitrito cobaltate solution:* A 5% w/v solution of sodium cobaltinitrite in water.

45. *Sodium hypochlorite solution:* A saturate solution of chlorine gas in 5% w/v solution of sodium hydroxide in water.

46. *Sodium tetrahydroxy stannate solution:* To 2 ml of 0.25 M stannous(II) chloride add 2 M sodium hydroxide solution with vigorous shaking, until the precipitate just dissolves. The reagent decomposes rapidly. Prepare fresh reagent when necessary.

47. *Stannous chloride solution:* A 1% w/v solution of stannous chloride in dilute hydrochloric acid.

48. *Starch iodide paper:* A filter paper dipped in starch solution and later in potassium iodide solution.

49. *Starch paper:* A filter paper dipped in 5% w/v solution of starch.

50. *Starch solution:* A 2% w/v solution of starch in water. Warm 100 ml of water and add 2 g of starch.

51. *Uranyl magnesium acetate reagent:* Dissolve 10 g Uranyl acetate dehydrate, in a mixture of 6 ml glacial acetic acid and 100 ml water (solution a). Dissolve 33 g of magnesium acetate tetra hydrate, in a mixture of 100 ml glacial acetic acid and 100 ml water (solution b). Mix the two solutions, allow to stand for 24 hours and filter.

7

General Monograph (A to Z) Assay Methods for Small Molecule Drugs

as per

Indian Pharmacopoeia-2014 and Addendum-2015

S. No	Title of Monograph	Assay method mentioned
1	Abacavir and Lamivudine Tablets	HPLC
2	Abacavir Oral Solution	HPLC
3	Abacavir Sulphate	HPLC
4	Abacavir Tablets	HPLC
5	Abacavir, Lamivudine and Zidovudine Tablets	HPLC
6	Absorbent Cotton	No assay mentioned
7	Absorbent Lint	No assay mentioned
8	Acamprosate Calcium	Acid-base titration
9	Acarbose	HPLC
10	Acarbose Tablets	HPLC
11	Acebutolol Hydrochloride	Acid-base titration
12	Acebutolol Tablets	UV spectroscopy
13	Aceclofenac	Acid-base titration
14	Aceclofenac Tablets	HPLC
15	Acepromazine Maleate	Non-Aqueous titration, $HClO_4$
16	Acesulphame Potassium	Non-Aqueous titration, $HClO_4$
17	Acetazolamide	Non-Aqueous titration, Tetrabutylammonium hydroxide

Contd...

S. No	Title of Monograph	Assay method mentioned
18	Acetazolamide Tablets	Non-Aqueous titration, Tetrabutylammonium hydroxide
19	Acetic acid ear drops	Acid-base titration
20	Aciclovir	Non-Aqueous titration, $HClO_4$
21	Aciclovir Cream	UV spectroscopy
22	Aciclovir dispersible tablets	UV spectroscopy
23	Aciclovir eye ointment	UV spectroscopy
24	Aciclovir intravenous infusion	UV spectroscopy
25	Aciclovir oral suspension	Fluorescence spectroscopy
26	Aciclovir tablets	UV spectroscopy
27	Acitretin	HPLC
28	Acitretin Capsules	HPLC
29	Activate Dimethicone	For polydimethylsiloxane-IR spectroscopy; for silicon dioxide-gravimetry
30	Activated Charcoal	No assay mentioned
31	Adefovir dipivoxil	Non-Aqueous titration, $HClO_4$
32	Adefovir tablets	HPLC
33	Adenosine	Non-Aqueous titration, $HClO_4$
34	Adenosine injection	HPLC
35	Adipic Acid	Acid-base titration
36	Adrenaline	Non-Aqueous titration, $HClO_4$
37	Adrenaline Injection	HPLC
38	Adrenaline tartrate	Non-Aqueous titration, $HClO_4$
39	Agomelatine	HPLC
40	Albendazole	Non-Aqueous titration, $HClO_4$
41	Albendazole oral suspension	HPLC
42	Albendazole tablets	UV spectroscopy
43	Alfacalcidol	HPLC
44	Alfacyclodextrin	HPLC
45	Alfuzosin hydrochloride	Non-Aqueous titration, $HClO_4$
46	Alfuzosin prolonged-release tablets	HPLC
47	Alfuzosin tablets	HPLC

Contd...

S. No	Title of Monograph	Assay method mentioned
48	Alginic acid	Acid-base titration
49	Allantoin	Acid-base titration
50	Allopurinol	Non-Aqueous titration, Tetrabutylammonium hydroxide
51	Allopurinol tablets	UV spectroscopy
52	Aloes	Visible spectroscopy
53	Alphamylase	Enzyme assay
54	Alprazolam	HPLC
55	Alprazolam prolonged release tablets	HPLC
56	Alprazolam tablets	HPLC
57	Alprostadil	HPLC
58	Alprostadil injection	HPLC
59	Aluminium Acetate Ear Drops	Complexometric titration
60	Aluminium hydroxide gel	Complexometric titration
61	Aluminium magnesium silicate	For Al-atomic absorption spectrometry, Mg-atomic absorption spectrometry
62	Amantadine Capsules	Non-Aqueous titration, $HClO_4$
63	Amantadine hydrochloride	Acid-base titration
64	Ambroxol Hydrochloride	Acid-base titration
65	Amikacin	Antibiotic assay
66	Amikacin Injection	Antibiotic assay
67	Amikacin Sulphate	Antibiotic assay
68	Amiloride hydrochloride	Non-Aqueous titration, $HClO_4$
69	Amiloride tablets	UV spectroscopy
70	Aminocaproic acid	Non-Aqueous titration, $HClO_4$
71	Aminocaproic acid injection	Non-Aqueous titration, $HClO_4$
72	Aminocaproic acid tablets	Non-Aqueous titration, $HClO_4$
73	Aminophylline (Theophylline, ethylene diamine)	For Theophylline-HPLC, Ethylenediamine-Acid-base titration
74	Aminophylline (Theophylline, ethylene diamine) injection	For Theophylline-HPLC, Ethylenediamine-Acid-base titration

Contd...

S. No	Title of Monograph	Assay method mentioned
75	Aminophylline (Theophylline, ethylene diamine) prolonged release tablets	For Theophylline-UV, Ethylene diamine-Acid-base titration
76	Aminophylline (Theophylline, ethylene diamine) tablets	For Theophylline-Argentometry titration, Ethylenediamine-Acid,base titration
77	Amiodarone hydrochloride	Acid-base titration
78	Amiodarone Intravenous Infusion	HPLC
79	Amiodarone tablets	HPLC
80	Amisulpride	Non-Aqueous titration, $HClO_4$
81	Amisulpride tablets	HPLC
82	Amitriptyline hydrochloride	HPLC
83	Amitriptyline hydrochloride tablets	HPLC
84	Amlodipine besylate	HPLC
85	Amlodipine besylate tablets	HPLC
86	Ammonium chloride	Acid-base titration
87	Amodiaquine hydrochloride	UV spectroscopy
88	Amodiaquine tablets	UV spectroscopy
89	Amorolifine hydrochloride	Non-Aqueous titration, $HClO_4$
90	Amoxcycillin and Potassium Clavulanate injection	HPLC
91	Amoxcycillin and Potassium Clavulanate oral suspension	HPLC
92	Amoxcycillin and Potassium Clavulanate tablets	HPLC
93	Amoxycillin capsules	HPLC
94	Amoxycillin dispersible tablets	HPLC
95	Amoxycillin injection	HPLC
96	Amoxycillin oral suspension	HPLC
97	Amoxycillin Sodium	HPLC
98	Amoxycillin trihydrate	HPLC
99	Amphotericin B	Assay of antibiotics
100	Amphotericin B injection	Assay of antibiotics
101	Ampicillin	HPLC

Contd...

S. No	Title of Monograph	Assay method mentioned
102	Ampicillin capsules	HPLC
103	Ampicillin dispersible tablets	HPLC
104	Ampicillin injection	HPLC
105	Ampicillin oral suspension	HPLC
106	Ampicillin sodium	HPLC
107	Ampicillin trihydrate	HPLC
108	Anastrozole	HPLC
109	Anastrozole tablets	HPLC
110	Anhydrous Lactose	No assay mentioned
111	Anticoagulant citrate dextrose solution	For Sodium citrate-Acid-base titration, Free citric acid-Acid-base titration, dextrose-optical rotation method
112	Anticoagulant citrate phosphate dextrose adenine solution	For total sodium-flame photometry/atomic absorption spectroscopy, for total citrate-visible spectroscopy, for dihydrogen phosphate dihydrate-Visible spectroscopy, for adenine-HPLC
113	Anticoagulant citrate phosphate dextrose solution	For Sodium citrate-Visible spectroscopy, free citric acid-Acid-base titration, Sodium dihydrogen phosphate dihydrate-Visible spectroscopy, dextrose-gravimetry
114	Aprotinin	Enzyme assay
115	Aqueous Calamine Cream	Gravimetry
116	Arbidol hydrochloride	HPLC
117	Arginine	Non-Aqueous titration, $HClO_4$
118	Aripiprazole	HPLC
119	Aripiprazole Tablets (Addendum-2015)	HPLC
120	Arteether	HPLC
121	Artemether	HPLC
122	Arterolane maleate	HPLC
123	Artesunate	HPLC
124	Ascorbic acid	Oxidation-Reduction titration (Iodimetry)

Contd...

S. No	Title of Monograph	Assay method mentioned
125	Ascorbic acid injection	Oxidation-reduction titration - 2,6 dichloro phenolindophenol
126	Ascorbic acid tablets	Oxidation-reduction titration (ceric)
127	Ascorbyl palmitate	Oxidation-Reduction titration (Iodimetry)
128	Asenapine maleate	HPLC
129	Aspartame	Non-Aqueous titration, $HClO_4$
130	Aspirin	Acid-base titration
131	Aspirin and Caffeine tablets	For Aspirin-Acid-base titration, for Caffeine-UV spectroscopy
132	Aspirin gastro resistant tablets	HPLC
133	Aspirin tablets	Acid-base titration
134	Atazanavir sulphate	HPLC
135	Atazanavir sulphate capsules	HPLC
136	Atenolol	Non-Aqueous titration, $HClO_4$
137	Atenolol tablets	UV spectroscopy
138	Atomoxetine hydrochloride	Non-Aqueous titration, $HClO_4$
139	Atorvastatin calcium	HPLC
140	Atorvastatin tablets	HPLC
141	Atosibane aceteate	HPLC
142	Atracurium besylate	HPLC
143	Atracurium besylate injection	HPLC
144	Atropine eye ointment	HPLC
145	Atropine injection	HPLC
146	Atropine Methonitrate	Non-Aqueous titration, $HClO_4$
147	Atropine sulphate	Non-Aqueous titration, $HClO_4$
148	Atropine tablets	HPLC
149	Azacitidine	HPLC
150	Azathioprine	Non-Aqueous titration, Tetrabutylammonium hydroxide
151	Azathioprine tablets	UV spectroscopy
152	Azelaic acid	Acid-base titration
153	Azelastine eye drops	HPLC
154	Azelastine hydrochloride	Non-Aqueous titration, $HClO_4$
155	Azelnidipine	HPLC

Contd...

S. No	Title of Monograph	Assay method mentioned
156	Azithromycin	HPLC
157	Azithromycin capsules	HPLC
158	Azithromycin oral suspension	HPLC
159	Azithromycin tablets	HPLC
160	Bacitracin	Assay of antibiotics
161	Bacitracin Zinc	Assay of antibiotics
162	Baclofen	Non-Aqueous titration, $HClO_4$
163	Baclofen oral solution	HPLC
164	Baclofen tablets	HPLC
165	Bambuterol hydrochloride	Acid-base titration
166	Bambuterol tablets	HPLC
167	Barium Sulphate	No assay mentioned
168	Barium Sulphate Oral Suspension (Addendum-2015)	Gravimetry
169	Barium sulphate suspension	Gravimetry
170	Beclomethasone dipropionate	HPLC
171	Beclomethasone inhalation	HPLC
172	Belomycin Injection	Antibiotic assay
173	Benazepril Hydrochloride	HPLC
174	Benazepril Hydrochloride Tablets	HPLC
175	Bentonite	No assay mentioned
176	Benzalkonium Chloride	Indicator extraction titration
177	Benzalkonium Chloride Solution	Indicator extraction titration
178	Benzathine Penicillin	HPLC
179	Benzathine Penicillin Injection	HPLC
180	Benzathine Penicillin Tablets	HPLC
181	Benzhexol Hydrochloride	Non-Aqueous titration, $HClO_4$
182	Benzhexol Tablets	HPLC
183	Benzocaine	Diazotisation titration (Nitrite titration)
184	Benzoic acid	Acid-base titration
185	Benzoic acid solution	Acid-base titration

Contd...

S. No	Title of Monograph	Assay Method Mentioned
186	Benzoin	Acid-base titration
187	Benzoyl Peroxide Cream	Oxidation-reduction titration (Iodometry)
188	Benzoyl Peroxide Gel	Oxidation-reduction titration (Iodometry)
189	Benzyl Alcohol	Acid-base titration
190	Benzyl Benzoate	Acid-base titration
191	Benzyl Benzoate Application	Acid-base titration
192	Benzylpenicillin Injection	HPLC
193	Benzylpenicillin Potassium	HPLC
194	Benzylpenicillin Sodium	HPLC
195	Betacyclodextrin	HPLC
196	Betahistine Hydrochloride	HPLC
197	Betahistine Mesylate	Non-Aqueous titration, $HClO_4$
198	Betahistine Tablets	HPLC
199	Betamethasone	UV spectroscopy
200	Betamethasone Cream	HPLC
201	Betamethasone Dipropionate	UV spectroscopy
202	Betamethasone Eye Drops	HPLC
203	Betamethasone Injection	UV spectroscopy
204	Betamethasone Lotion	HPLC
205	Betamethasone Ointment	HPLC
206	Betamethasone Sodium Phosphate	UV spectroscopy
207	Betamethasone Sodium Phosphate Tablets	HPLC
208	Betamethasone Tablets	HPLC
209	Betamethasone Valerate	HPLC
210	Betamethasone Valerate Cream	HPLC
211	Betamethasone Valerate Ointment	HPLC
212	Betaxolol Eye Drops	HPLC
213	Betaxolol Hydrochloride	Acid-base titration
214	Bezafibrate	Acid-base titration
215	Bezafibrate Tablets	UV spectroscopy

Contd...

S. No	Title of Monograph	Assay Method Mentioned
216	Biapenem	HPLC
217	Bicalutamide	HPLC
218	Bicalutamide Tablets	HPLC
219	Bifonazole	Non-Aqueous titration, $HClO_4$
220	Bifonazole Cream	HPLC
221	Biperiden Hydrochloride	Non-Aqueous titration, $HClO_4$
222	Biperiden Tablets	UV spectroscopy
223	Biphasic Insulin Aspart Injection	HPLC
224	Biphasic Insulin Injection	Assay of Insulin
225	Biphasic Insulin Lispro Injection	HPLC
226	Biphasic Isophane Insulin Injection	Assay of Insulin
227	Bisacodyl	Non-Aqueous titration, $HClO_4$
228	Bisacodyl Gastro-resistant Tablets	HPLC
229	Bisacodyl Suppositories	Non-Aqueous titration, $HClO_4$
230	Bismuth Subcarbonate	Complexometric titration
231	Bleomycin Sulphate	Antibiotic assay
232	Boric Acid	Acid-base titration
233	Bortezomib	HPLC
234	Brimonidine Tartrate (Addendum-2015)	Non-Aqueous titration, $HClO_4$
235	Brimonidine Tartrate Eye Drops (Addendum-2015)	HPLC
236	Brinzolamide	HPLC
237	Brinzolamide Ophthalmic Suspension (Addendum-2015)	HPLC
238	Bromhexine Hydrochloride	Acid-base titration
239	Bromhexine Tablets	UV spectroscopy
240	Bromocriptine Capsules	UV spectroscopy
241	Bromocriptine Mesylate	Non-Aqueous titration, $HClO_4$
242	Bromocriptine Tablets	UV spectroscopy
243	Bronopol	Argentometry titration (Volhard method)
244	Buclizine Hydrochloride	Non-Aqueous titration, $HClO_4$

Contd...

S. No	Title of Monograph	Assay Method Mentioned
245	Budesonide	HPLC
246	Budesonide Inhalation (Addendum-2015)	HPLC
247	Budesonide Powder for Inhalation (Addendum-2015)	HPLC
248	Bumetanide	Acid-base titration
249	Bumetanide Injection	HPLC
250	Bumetanide Oral Solution	HPLC
251	Bumetanide Tablets	HPLC
252	Bupivacaine Hydrochloride	Acid-base titration
253	Bupivacaine Injection	HPLC
254	Buprenorphine Hydrochloride	Non-Aqueous titration, $HClO_4$
255	Buprenorphine Injection	Visible spectroscopy
256	Buprenorphine Tablets	Visible spectroscopy
257	Buspirone Hydrochloride	Non-Aqueous titration, $HClO_4$
258	Buspirone Tablets	HPLC
259	Busulphan	Acid-base titration
260	Busulphan Tablets	Gas Chromatography
261	Butylated Hydroxytoluene	No assay mentioned
262	Butylparaben	HPLC
263	Cabergoline	HPLC
264	Cabergoline Tablets	HPLC
265	Caffeine	Non-Aqueous titration, $HClO_4$
266	Caffeine Citrate Oral Solution	HPLC
267	Calamine	Acid-base titration
268	Calamine Lotion	No assay mentioned
269	Calamine Ointment	Gravimetry
270	Calcipotriol Anhydrous	HPLC
271	Calcipotriol Ointment	HPLC
272	Calcitonin (Salmon)	HPLC
273	Calcitonin (Salmon) Injection	HPLC
274	Calcitriol	HPLC
275	Calcitriol Capsules	HPLC
276	Calcium Carbonate	Complexometric titration

Contd...

S. No	Title of Monograph	Assay Method Mentioned
277	Calcium Carbonate Tablets	Complexometric titration
278	Calcium Chloride	Complexometric titration
279	Calcium Chloride Injection	Complexometric titration
280	Calcium Dobesilate Monohydrate	Oxidation-reduction titration (ceric)
281	Calcium Folinate	HPLC
282	Calcium Folinate Injection	HPLC
283	Calcium Gluconate	Complexometric titration
284	Calcium Gluconate Injection	Complexometric titration
285	Calcium Gluconate Tablets	Complexometric titration
286	Calcium Lactate	Complexometric titration
287	Calcium Lactate Tablets	Complexometric titration
288	Calcium Levulinate	Complexometric titration
289	Calcium Levulinate Injection	Complexometric titration
290	Calcium Panthothenate	Non-Aqueous titration, $HClO_4$
291	Calcium Panthothenate Tablets (Addendum-2015)	HPLC
292	Calcium stearate	Complexometric titration
293	Capecitabine	HPLC
294	Capecitabine Tablets	HPLC
295	Capreomycin Injection	Antibiotic assay
296	Capreomycin Sulphate	Antibiotic assay
297	Captopril	Oxidation-Reduction titration (Iodate titration, Iodometry titration)
298	Captopril Tablets	HPLC
299	Carbamazepine	HPLC
300	Carbamazepine Prolonged-release Tablets	HPLC
301	Carbamazepine Tablets	HPLC
302	Carbenicillin Sodium	Antibiotic assay
303	Carbenicillin Sodium Injection	Antibiotic assay
304	Carbenoxolone Sodium	Non-Aqueous titration, Tetrabutylammonium hydroxide
305	Carbenoxolone Sodium Tablets	UV spectroscopy
306	Carbidopa	Non-Aqueous titration, $HClO_4$

Contd...

S. No	Title of Monograph	Assay Method Mentioned
307	Carbimazole	UV spectroscopy
308	Carbimazole Tablets	UV spectroscopy
309	Carbomers	Acid-base titration
310	Carboplatin	Gravimetry
311	Carboplatin Injection	HPLC
312	Carboprost Tromethamine	HPLC
313	Carboprost Tromethamine Injection	HPLC
314	Carboxymethylcellulose Calcium	No assay mentioned
315	Carboxymethylcellulose Eye Drops	UV spectroscopy
316	Carboxymethylcellulose Sodium	Non-Aqueous titration, $HClO_4$
317	Carisoprodol	Acid-base titration
318	Carisoprodol Tablets	HPLC
319	Carnauba Wax	No assay mentioned
320	Carvedilol	Non-Aqueous titration, $HClO_4$
321	Carvedilol Tablets	HPLC
322	Cefaclor	HPLC
323	Cefaclor Capsules	HPLC
324	Cefaclor Oral Suspension	HPLC
325	Cefaclor Prolonged-release Tablets	HPLC
326	Cefadroxil	HPLC
327	Cefadroxil Capsules	HPLC
328	Cefadroxil Oral Suspension	HPLC
329	Cefadroxil Tablets	HPLC
330	Cefamandole Injection	HPLC
331	Cefamandole Nafate	HPLC
332	Cefazolin Sodium	HPLC
333	Cefazolin Sodium Injection	HPLC
334	Cefepime Hydrochloride	HPLC
335	Cefepime Injection	HPLC
336	Cefixime	HPLC
337	Cefixime Oral Suspension	HPLC

Contd...

S. No	Title of Monograph	Assay Method Mentioned
338	Cefixime Tablets	HPLC
339	Cefoperazone Injection	HPLC
340	Cefoperazone Sodium	HPLC
341	Cefotaxime Sodium	HPLC
342	Cefotaxime Sodium Injection	HPLC
343	Cefpirome Injection	HPLC
344	Cefpirome Sulphate	HPLC
345	Cefpodoxime Oral Suspension	HPLC
346	Cefpodoxime Proxetil	HPLC
347	Cefpodoxime Tablets	HPLC
348	Ceftazidime	HPLC
349	Ceftazidime for Injection	HPLC
350	Ceftazidime Injection	HPLC
351	Ceftiofur Sodium	HPLC
352	Ceftriaxone Injection	HPLC
353	Ceftriaxone Sodium	HPLC
354	Cefuroxime Axetil	HPLC
355	Cefuroxime Axetil Tablets	HPLC
356	Cefuroxime Injection	HPLC
357	Cefuroxime Sodium	HPLC
358	Celiprolol Hydrochloride	Acid-base titration
359	Celiprolol Tablets	HPLC
360	Cellulose Acetate Phthalate	For acetyl groups-Acid-base titration; for hydrogen phthaloyl groups-Acid-base titration
361	Cephalexin	HPLC
362	Cephalexin Capsules	HPLC
363	Cephalexin Oral Suspension	HPLC
364	Cephalexin Tablets	HPLC
365	Cephaloridine	Oxidation-Reduction titration (Iodimetry)
366	Cephaloridine Injection	Oxidation-Reduction titration (Iodimetry)
367	Cetirizine Hydrochloride	Acid-base titration
368	Cetirizine Syrup	HPLC

Contd...

S. No	Title of Monograph	Assay Method Mentioned
369	Cetirizine Tablets	HPLC
370	Cetostearyl Alcohol	Gas Chromatography
371	Cetrimide	Oxidation-reduction titration (Iodate titration)
372	Cetrimide Cream	Indicator extraction titration
373	Cetrimide Emulsifying Ointment	Indicator extraction titration
374	Cetyl Alcohol	Gas Chromatography
375	Cetyl Palmitate	Gas Chromatography
376	Chlorambucil	Acid-base titration
377	Chlorambucil Tablets	HPLC
378	Chloramphenicol	UV spectroscopy
379	Chloramphenicol Capsules	UV spectroscopy
380	Chloramphenicol Ear Drops	HPLC
381	Chloramphenicol Eye Drops	HPLC
382	Chloramphenicol Eye Ointment	HPLC
383	Chloramphenicol Oral Suspension	UV spectroscopy
384	Chloramphenicol Palmitate	UV spectroscopy
385	Chloramphenicol Sodium Succinate	UV spectroscopy
386	Chloramphenicol Sodium Succinate Injection	UV spectroscopy
387	Chlorbutol	Argentometry titration (Volhard method)
388	Chlorcyclizine Hydrochloride	Acid-base titration
389	Chlordiazepoxide	Non-Aqueous titration, $HClO_4$
390	Chlordiazepoxide Tablets	UV spectroscopy
391	Chlorhexidine Acetate	Non-Aqueous titration, $HClO_4$
392	Chlorhexidine Gluconate Solution	Non-Aqueous titration, $HClO_4$
393	Chlorhexidine Hydrochloride	Non-Aqueous titration, $HClO_4$
394	Chlorhexidine Mouthwash	HPLC
395	Chlorocresol	Oxidation-Reduction (Iodometry)
396	Chloroform	No assay mentioned

Contd...

S. No	Title of Monograph	Assay Method Mentioned
397	Chloroquine Phosphate	HPLC
398	Chloroquine Phosphate Injection	Non-Aqueous titration, $HClO_4$
399	Chloroquine Phosphate Suspension	UV spectroscopy
400	Chloroquine Phosphate Tablets	HPLC
401	Chloroquine Sulphate	Non-Aqueous titration, $HClO_4$
402	Chloroquine Sulphate Injection	Non-Aqueous titration, $HClO_4$
403	Chloroquine Sulphate Tablets	Non-Aqueous titration, $HClO_4$
404	Chloroquine Syrup	Non-Aqueous titration, $HClO_4$
405	Chlorothiazide	Non-Aqueous titration, Tetrabutylammonium hydroxide
406	Chlorothiazide Oral Suspension	UV spectroscopy
407	Chlorothiazide Tablets	HPLC
408	Chloroxylenol	Oxidation-Reduction titration (Iodometry)
409	Chloroxylenol solution	Gas Chromatography
410	Chlorpheniramine Injection	UV spectroscopy
411	Chlorpheniramine Maleate	Non-Aqueous titration, $HClO_4$
412	Chlorpheniramine Tablets	UV spectroscopy
413	Chlorpromazine Hydrochloride	Non-Aqueous titration, $HClO_4$
414	Chlorpromazine Injection	UV spectroscopy
415	Chlorpromazine Tablets	UV spectroscopy
416	Chlorpropamide	Acid-base titration
417	Chlorpropamide Tablets	UV spectroscopy
418	Chlorthalidone	Non-Aqueous titration, Tetrabutylammonium hydroxide
419	Chlorthalidone Tablets	UV spectroscopy
420	Cholecalciferol	HPLC
421	Cholecalciferol Injection	Visible spectroscopy
422	Cholecalciferol Tablets	HPLC
423	Choline Fenofibrate	For Fenofibric acid-HPLC, for Choline-Non-Aqueous titration, $HClO_4$

Contd...

S. No	Title of Monograph	Assay Method Mentioned
424	Chorionic Gonadotrophin	Biological assay
425	Chorionic Gonadotrophin Injection	Biological assay
426	Chymotrypsin	Enzyme assay
427	Ciclesonide	HPLC
428	Ciclesonide Inhalation	HPLC
429	Cilastatin Sodium	HPLC
430	Cilostazol	HPLC
431	Cilostazol Tablets	HPLC
432	Cimetidine	Non-Aqueous titration, $HClO_4$
433	Cimetidine Tablets	Non-Aqueous titration, $HClO_4$
434	Cinnarizine	Non-Aqueous titration, $HClO_4$
435	Cinnarizine Tablets	HPLC
436	Ciprofloxacin	HPLC
437	Ciprofloxacin Eye Drops	HPLC
438	Ciprofloxacin Hydrochloride	HPLC
439	Ciprofloxacin Injection	HPLC
440	Ciprofloxacin Tablets	HPLC
441	Cisplatin	HPLC
442	Cisplatin Injection	HPLC
443	Citalopram Hydrobromide	HPLC
444	Citalopram Tablets	HPLC
445	Citicoline Injection (Addendum-2015)	HPLC
446	Citicoline Prolonged-release Tablets (Addendum-2015)	HPLC
447	Citicoline Sodium	HPLC
448	Citicoline Tablets (Addendum-2015)	HPLC
449	Citric Acid	Acid-base titration
450	Citric Acid Monohydrate	Acid-base titration
451	Clarithromycin	HPLC
452	Clarithromycin Tablets	HPLC
453	Clemastine Fumarate	Non-Aqueous titration, $HClO_4$
454	Clemastine Oral Solution (Addendum-2015)	HPLC

Contd...

S. No	Title of Monograph	Assay Method Mentioned
455	Clemastine Tablets	HPLC
456	Clindamycin Capsules	HPLC
457	Clindamycin Hydrochloride	HPLC
458	Clindamycin Injection	HPLC
459	Clindamycin Phosphate	HPLC
460	Clobazam	UV spectroscopy
461	Clobazam Capsules	HPLC
462	Clobetasol Cream	HPLC
463	Clobetasol Ointment	HPLC
464	Clobetasol Propionate	HPLC
465	Clobetasone Butyrate	UV spectroscopy
466	Clobetasone Cream	HPLC
467	Clofazimine	Non-Aqueous titration, $HClO_4$
468	Clofazimine Capsules	Visible spectroscopy
469	Clomifene Citrate	Non-Aqueous titration, $HClO_4$
470	Clomifene Tablets	UV spectroscopy
471	Clomipramine Capsules	HPLC
472	Clomipramine Hydrochloride	Acid-base titration
473	Clonazepam	Non-Aqueous titration, $HClO_4$
474	Clonazepam Injection	UV spectroscopy
475	Clonazepam Tablets	HPLC
476	Clonidine Hydrochloride	Acid-base titration
477	Clonidine Injection	Visible spectroscopy
478	Clonidine Tablets	Visible spectroscopy
479	Clopidogrel Bisulphate	HPLC
480	Clopidogrel Tablets	HPLC
481	Clotrimazole	Non-Aqueous titration, $HClO_4$
482	Clotrimazole Cream	HPLC
483	Clotrimazole Pessaries	HPLC
484	Cloxacillin Capsules	HPLC
485	Cloxacillin Injection	HPLC
486	Cloxacillin Sodium	HPLC
487	Cloxacillin Syrup	HPLC
488	Clozapine	Non-Aqueous titration, $HClO_4$
489	Clozapine Tablets	HPLC

Contd...

S. No	Title of Monograph	Assay Method Mentioned
490	Codeine Phosphate	Non-Aqueous titration, $HClO_4$
491	Codeine Syrup	Acid-base titration
492	Codeine Tablets	Acid-base titration
493	Colchicine	Non-Aqueous titration, $HClO_4$
494	Colchicine and Probenecid Tablets	For Colchicine- UV spectroscopy, for probenecid-UV spectroscopy
495	Colchicine Tablets	HPLC
496	Colistimethate Injection	Antibiotic assay
497	Colistimethate Sodium	Antibiotic assay
498	Colistin Sulphate	HPLC
499	Colistin Tablets	Antibiotic assay
500	Colloidal Silicon Dioxide	Gravimetry
501	Compound Benzoic acid ointment	For Benzoic acid-Acid-base titration; for salicylic acid-Visible spectroscopy
502	Compound Benzoin Tincture	Acid-base titration
503	Compound Sodium Chloride and Dextrose Injection	For Sodium chloride-Flame photometry or Atomic Absorption Spectrometry; for Potassium chloride-Flame photometry or Atomic Absorption Spectrometry; for Calcium chloride-Complexometry titration; for total chloride-Argentometry (Volhard's method); for dextrose-Optical rotation
504	Compound Sodium Chloride Injection	For Sodium chloride-Flame photometry or Atomic Absorption Spectrometry; for Potassium chloride-Flame photometry or Atomic Absorption Spectrometry; for Calcium chloride-Complexometry titration
505	Compound Sodium Chloride Solution	For Sodium chloride-Flame photometry or Atomic Absorption Spectrometry; for Potassium chloride-Flame photometry or Atomic Absorption Spectrometry; for Calcium chloride-Complexometry titration

Contd...

S. No	Title of Monograph	Assay Method Mentioned
506	Compound Sodium Lactate and Dextrose Injection	For Sodium-Flame photometry or Atomic Absorption Spectrometry; for Potassium-Flame photometry or Atomic Absorption Spectrometry; for total chlorides-Argentometry (Volhard's method); for calcium chloride-Complexometry titration; for lactate-HPLC; for dextrose-Optical rotation
507	Compound Sodium Lactate Injection	For Sodium-Flame photometry or Atomic Absorption Spectrometry; for Potassium-Flame photometry or Atomic Absorption Spectrometry; for total chlorides-Argentometry (Volhard's method); for calcium chloride-Complexometry titration; for lactate-Acid-base titration
508	Compound Sodium Lactate Solution and Irrigation	For Sodium-Flame photometry or Atomic Absorption Spectrometry; for Potassium-Flame photometry or Atomic Absorption Spectrometry; for total chlorides-Argentometry (Volhard's method); for calcium chloride-Complexometry titration; for lactate-HPLC
509	Concentrated Vitamin D Solution	Column chromatography and Visible spectroscopy
510	Concentrated Vitamins A and D Solution	For vitamin A-UV spectroscopy; for vitamin D-Column chromatography and visible spectroscopy
511	Corn Oil	No assay mentioned
512	Cortisone Acetate	UV spectroscopy
513	Cortisone Injection	HPLC
514	Cortisone Tablets	HPLC
515	Cottonseed Oil	No assay mentioned
516	Cresol	No assay mentioned

Contd...

S. No	Title of Monograph	Assay Method Mentioned
517	Cresol with Soap Solution	Gravimetry
518	Croscarmellose Sodium	No assay mentioned
519	Crospovidone	No assay mentioned
520	Crotamiton	HPLC
521	Crotamiton Cream	HPLC
522	Cyanocobalamin	UV spectroscopy
523	Cyanocobalamin Injection	UV spectroscopy
524	Cyclizine Hydrochloride	Non-Aqueous titration, $HClO_4$
525	Cyclizine Tablets	UV spectroscopy
526	Cyclopentolate Eye Drops	HPLC
527	Cyclopentolate Hydrochloride	Acid-base titration
528	Cyclophosphamide	Argentometry titration (Volhard method)
529	Cyclophosphamide Injection	HPLC
530	Cyclophosphamide Tablets	Argentometry titration (Volhard method)
531	Cycloserine	HPLC
532	Cycloserine Capsules	HPLC
533	Cycloserine Tablets	Visible spectroscopy
534	Cyclosporine	HPLC
535	Cyclosporine Capsules	HPLC
536	Cyproheptadine Hydrochloride	Non-Aqueous titration, $HClO_4$
537	Cyproheptadine Syrup	UV spectroscopy
538	Cyproheptadine Tablets	UV spectroscopy
539	Cyproterone Acetate	UV spectroscopy
540	Cyproterone Tablets	HPLC
541	Cytarabine	Non-Aqueous titration, $HClO_4$
542	Cytarabine Injection	Non-Aqueous titration, $HClO_4$
543	Dalteparin Sodium	No assay mentioned
544	Dalteparin Sodium Injection	Anti-factor Xa activity, and Xa to IIa ratio
545	Danazol	UV spectroscopy
546	Danazol Capsules	HPLC
547	Dapoxetine Hydrochloride	HPLC

Contd...

S. No	Title of Monograph	Assay Method Mentioned
548	Dapsone	Diazotisation titration (Nitrite titration)
549	Dapsone Tablets	Diazotisation titration (Nitrite titration)
550	Daunorubicin Hydrochloride	HPLC
551	Daunorubicin Injection	HPLC
552	Dehydroacetic Acid	Acid-base titration
553	Dehydroemetine Hydrochloride	Non-Aqueous titration, $HClO_4$
554	Dehydroemetine Injection	UV spectroscopy
555	Dequalinium Chloride	Non-Aqueous titration, $HClO_4$
556	Desferrioxamine Injection	Visible spectroscopy
557	Desferrioxamine Mesylate	Visible spectroscopy
558	Desmopressin	HPLC
559	Desmopressin Intranasal Solution	HPLC
560	Desoxycortone Acetate	UV spectroscopy
561	Desoxycortone Acetate Injection	UV spectroscopy
562	Dexamethasone	UV spectroscopy
563	Dexamethasone Injection	HPLC
564	Dexamethasone Sodium Phosphate	UV spectroscopy
565	Dexamethasone Tablets	HPLC
566	Dexchlorpheniramine Maleate	Non-Aqueous titration, $HClO_4$
567	Dexchlorpheniramine Oral Solution	UV spectroscopy
568	Dexchlorpheniramine Tablets	UV spectroscopy
569	Dexlansoprazole	HPLC
570	Dextran 110 Injection	Optical rotation
571	Dextran 40 Injection	Optical rotation
572	Dextran 70 Injection	Optical rotation
573	Dextrin	No assay mentioned
574	Dextromethorphan Hydrobromide	Acid-base titration
575	Dextromethorphan Hydrobromide Syrup	HPLC

Contd...

S. No	Title of Monograph	Assay Method Mentioned
576	Dextropropoxyphene Capsules	Non-Aqueous titration, $HClO_4$
577	Dextropropoxyphene Hydrochloride	Non-Aqueous titration, $HClO_4$
578	Dextropropoxyphene Napsilate	Non-Aqueous titration, $HClO_4$
579	Dextrose	No assay mentioned
580	Dextrose Injection	Optical rotation
581	Diacerein	HPLC
582	Diacerein Capsules	HPLC
583	Diazepam	Non-Aqueous titration, $HClO_4$
584	Diazepam Capsules	UV spectroscopy
585	Diazepam Injection	UV spectroscopy
586	Diazepam Tablets	UV spectroscopy
587	Diazoxide	Acid-base titration
588	Diazoxide Tablets	UV spectroscopy
589	Dibasic Calcium Phosphate	Complexometric titration
590	Diclofenac Gastro-resistant Tablets	HPLC
591	Diclofenac Injection	HPLC
592	Diclofenac Prolonged-release Tablets	HPLC
593	Diclofenac Sodium	Non-Aqueous titration, $HClO_4$
594	Dicloxacillin Capsules	HPLC
595	Dicloxacillin Oral Suspension	HPLC
596	Dicloxacillin Sodium	HPLC
597	Dicyclomine Hydrochloride	Non-Aqueous titration, $HClO_4$
598	Dicyclomine Injection	HPLC
599	Dicyclomine Oral Solution	Indicator extraction titration
600	Dicyclomine Tablets	Indicator extraction titration
601	Didanosine	HPLC
602	Didanosine Gastro-resistant Capsules	HPLC
603	Didanosine Tablets	HPLC
604	Dienoestrol	UV spectroscopy
605	Dienoestrol Tablets	UV spectroscopy

Contd...

S. No	Title of Monograph	Assay Method Mentioned
606	Dienogest	HPLC
607	Diethanolamine	Acid-base titration
608	Diethyl Phthalate	Acid-base titration
609	Diethylcarbamazine Citrate	HPLC
610	Diethylcarbamazine Tablets	HPLC
611	Diethylphenylacetamide	Gas Chromatography
612	Diethyltoluamide	Acid-base titration
613	Digitoxin	Visible spectroscopy
614	Digitoxin Tablets	Visible spectroscopy
615	Digoxin	HPLC
616	Digoxin Injection	Visible spectroscopy
617	Digoxin Paediatric Solution	Visible spectroscopy
618	Digoxin Tablets	Visible spectroscopy
619	Dihydroergocristine Mesylate	Non-Aqueous titration, Tetrabutylammonium hydroxide
620	Dihydroergotamine Mesylate	Non-Aqueous titration, $HClO_4$
621	Diiodohydroxyquinoline	Non-Aqueous titration, Tetrabutylammonium hydroxide
622	Diiodohydroxyquinoline Tablets	Oxidation-reduction titration (Oxygen flask method-Iodometry)
623	Diloxanide Furoate	Non-Aqueous titration, Tetrabutylammonium hydroxide
624	Diloxanide Tablets	UV spectroscopy
625	Diltiazem Hydrochloride	HPLC
626	Diltiazem Injection	HPLC
627	Diltiazem Tablets	HPLC
628	Dilute Hydrochloric acid	Acid-base titration
629	Diluted Glyceryl Trinitrate	HPLC
630	Diluted Isosorbide Dinitrate	HPLC
631	Diluted Isosorbide Mononitrate	HPLC
632	Diluted Pentaerythritol Tetranitrate	HPLC
633	Dimercaprol	Oxidation-Reduction titration (Iodimetry)
634	Dimercaprol Injection	Oxidation-Reduction titration (Iodimetry)

Contd...

S. No	Title of Monograph	Assay Method Mentioned
635	Dimethicone	IR spectroscopy
636	Diphenhydramine Capsules	Acid-base titration
637	Diphenhydramine Hydrochloride	Acid-base titration
638	Diphenoxylate Hydrochloride	Acid-base titration
639	Dipivefrine Eye Drops	HPLC
640	Dipivefrine Hydrochloride	HPLC
641	Dipyridamole	Non-Aqueous titration, $HClO_4$
642	Dipyridamole Tablets	UV spectroscopy
643	Disodium Edetate	Complexometric titration
644	Disodium Edetate Injection	Complexometric titration
645	Disopyramide	Non-Aqueous titration, $HClO_4$
646	Disopyramide Capsules	UV spectroscopy
647	Disopyramide Phosphate Capsules	UV spectroscopy
648	Disopyramide Phosphate Prolonged-release Capsules	UV spectroscopy
649	Disulfiram	Argentometry titration
650	Disulfiram Tablets	Visible spectroscopy
651	Dithranol	Non-Aqueous titration, Tetrabutylammonium hydroxide
652	Dithranol Ointment	HPLC
653	Divalproex Gastro-resistant Tablets	HPLC
654	Divalproex Prolonged-release Tablets	HPLC
655	Divalproex Sodium	HPLC
656	Dobutamine Hydrochloride	HPLC
657	Dobutamine Injection	HPLC
658	Docetaxel Anhydrous	HPLC
659	Docetaxel Injection	HPLC
660	Docetaxel Trihydrate	HPLC
661	Docusate Sodium	Acid-base titration
662	Docusate Tablets	HPLC
663	Domperidone	Non-Aqueous titration, $HClO_4$
664	Domperidone Maleate	Non-Aqueous titration, $HClO_4$

Contd...

S. No	Title of Monograph	Assay Method Mentioned
665	Domperidone Suspension	HPLC
666	Donepezil Hydrochloride	Non-Aqueous titration, $HClO_4$
667	Donepezil Tablets	HPLC
668	Dopamine Hydrochloride	Non-Aqueous titration, $HClO_4$
669	Dopamine Injection	HPLC
670	Dorzolamide and Timolol Eye Drops (Addendum-2015)	For Dorzolamide-HPLC; Timolol-HPLC
671	Dorzolamide Hydrochloride (Addendum-2015)	HPLC
672	Dothiepin Capsules	Non-Aqueous titration, $HClO_4$
673	Dothiepin Hydrochloride	Non-Aqueous titration, $HClO_4$
674	Doxapram Hydrochloride	Acid-base titration
675	Doxapram Injection	UV spectroscopy
676	Doxepin Capsules	UV spectroscopy
677	Doxepin Hydrochloride	Non-Aqueous titration, $HClO_4$
678	Doxofylline	HPLC
679	Doxofylline Tablets	HPLC
680	Doxorubicin Hydrochloride	HPLC
681	Doxorubicin Injection	HPLC
682	Doxycycline Capsules	HPLC
683	Doxycycline Hydrochloride	HPLC
684	D-Panthenol	Acid-base titration
685	Dried Aluminium hydroxide	Complexometric titration
686	Dried Ferrous Sulphate	Oxidation-reduction titration (ceric)
687	Drotaverine Tablets	HPLC
688	Dutasteride	HPLC
689	Dutasteride Capsules (Addendum-2015)	HPLC
690	Dydrogesterone	HPLC
691	Dydrogesterone Tablets	HPLC
692	Ebastine	Non-Aqueous titration, $HClO_4$
693	Ebastine Tablets (Addendum-2015)	HPLC
694	Eberconazole Nitrate	HPLC
695	Econazole Cream	Gas Chromatography
696	Econazole Nitrate	Non-Aqueous titration, $HClO_4$

Contd...

S. No	Title of Monograph	Assay Method Mentioned
697	Econazole Pessaries	Non-Aqueous titration, $HClO_4$
698	Efavirenz	HPLC
699	Efavirenz Capsules	HPLC
700	Efavirenz Tablets	HPLC
701	Efavirenz, Emitricitabine and Tenofovir Tablets	HPLC
702	Eletriptan Hydrobromide	HPLC
703	Emtricitabine	HPLC
704	Emtricitabine Capsules	HPLC
705	Emulsifying Wax	No assay mentioned
706	Enalapril Maleate	HPLC
707	Enalapril Maleate Tablets	HPLC
708	Enoxaparin Injection	Anti-factor Xa activity, and Xa to IIa ratio
709	Enoxaparin Sodium	Anti-factor Xa activity, and Xa to IIa ratio
710	Entacapone	HPLC
711	Entacapone Tablets (Addendum-2015)	HPLC
712	Ephedrine Hydrochloride	Non-Aqueous titration, $HClO_4$
713	Ephedrine Nasal Drops	HPLC
714	Ephedrine Oral Solution	HPLC
715	Ephedrine Tablets	HPLC
716	Epinastine Eye Drops	HPLC
717	Epinastine Hydrochloride	Non-Aqueous titration, $HClO_4$
718	Eplerenone	HPLC
719	Eptifibatide	HPLC
720	Eptifibatide Injection	HPLC
721	Ergocalciferol	HPLC
722	Ergocalciferol Tablets	HPLC
723	Ergometrine Injection	Visible spectroscopy
724	Ergometrine Maleate	Non-Aqueous titration, $HClO_4$
725	Ergometrine Tablets	Visible spectroscopy
726	Ergotamine Injection	Visible spectroscopy
727	Ergotamine Tablets	Visible spectroscopy
728	Ergotamine Tartrate	Non-Aqueous titration, $HClO_4$
729	Erlotinib Hydrochloride	HPLC

Contd...

S. No	Title of Monograph	Assay Method Mentioned
730	Erlotinib Tablets	HPLC
731	Erythormycin Gastro-resistant tablets	Antibiotic assay
732	Erythromycin	Antibiotic assay
733	Erythromycin Stearate	Antibiotic assay
734	Erythromycin Stearate Tablets	Antibiotic assay
735	Escitalopram Oxalate	HPLC
736	Escitalopram Tablets	HPLC
737	Eslicarbazepine Acetate	HPLC
738	Eslicarbazepine Tablets (Addendum-2015)	HPLC
739	Esmolol Hydrochloride	HPLC
740	Esomeprazole Gastro-resistant Tablets	HPLC
741	Esomeprazole Magnesium Trihydrate	HPLC
742	Estradiol and Norethisterone Tablets	HPLC
743	Ethacrynic Acid	Acid-base titration
744	Ethacrynic Acid Tablets	HPLC
745	Ethambutol and Isoniazid Tablets	For Isoniazid-HPLC; for Ethambutol Hydrochloride-HPLC
746	Ethambutol Hydrochloride	HPLC
747	Ethambutol Injection	HPLC
748	Ethambutol Tablets	HPLC
749	Ethanol	Relative density
750	Ethanol (95 percent)	Relative density
751	Ethanolamine	Acid-base titration
752	Ethinyloestradiol	Acid-base titration
753	Ethinyloestradiol Tablets	HPLC
754	Ethionamide	HPLC
755	Ethionamide Tablets	HPLC
756	Ethopropazine Hydrochloride	Non-Aqueous titration, $HClO_4$
757	Ethopropazine Tablets	UV spectroscopy
758	Ethosuximide	Non-Aqueous titration, Tetrabutylammonium hydroxide

Contd...

S. No	Title of Monograph	Assay Method Mentioned
759	Ethosuximide Capsules	Non-Aqueous titration, Tetrabutylammonium hydroxide
760	Ethosuximide Syrup	Gas Chromatography
761	Ethyl Chloride	No assay mentioned
762	Ethyl Oleate	Acid-base titration
763	Ethyl Vanillin	Non-Aqueous titration, (Sodium methoxide)
764	Ethylcellulose	Oxidation-redution titration (Iodometry-methoxyl determination)
765	Ethylenediamine Hydrate	Acid-base titration
766	Ethyloestrenol	Gas Chromatography
767	Ethyloestrenol Tablets	Gas Chromatography
768	Ethylparaben	HPLC
769	Etidronate Disodium	Non-Aqueous titration, $HClO_4$
770	Etidronate Tablets	HPLC
771	Etodolac	Non-Aqueous titration, Tetrabutylammonium hydroxide
772	Etodolac Capsules	HPLC
773	Etodolac Tablets	HPLC
774	Etophylline and Theophylline Prolonged-release Tablets	HPLC
775	Etoposide	HPLC
776	Etoposide Capsules	HPLC
777	Etoposide Injection	HPLC
778	Etoricoxib	HPLC
779	Etoricoxib Tablets	HPLC
780	Ezetimibe	HPLC
781	Ezetimibe Tablets	HPLC
782	Famciclovir	HPLC
783	Famciclovir Tablets	HPLC
784	Famotidine	Non-Aqueous titration, $HClO_4$
785	Famotidine Tablets	HPLC
786	Fasoterodine Fumarate	HPLC
787	Fasudil Hydrochloride	Non-Aqueous titration, $HClO_4$
788	Felodipine	Oxidation-reduction titration

Contd...

S. No	Title of Monograph	Assay Method Mentioned
789	Felodipine Prolonged-release Tablets	HPLC
790	Fenbendazole	Non-Aqueous titration, $HClO_4$
791	Fenofibrate	HPLC
792	Fenofibrate Capsules	HPLC
793	Fenspiride Hydrochloride	Non-Aqueous titration, $HClO_4$
794	Fentanyl	Non-Aqueous titration, $HClO_4$
795	Fentanyl Citrate	Non-Aqueous titration, $HClO_4$
796	Fentanyl Injection	HPLC
797	Ferrous Fumarate	Oxidation-reduction titration (ceric)
798	Ferrous Fumarate Tablets	Oxidation-reduction titration (ceric)
799	Ferrous Gluconate	Oxidation-reduction titration (ceric)
800	Ferrous Gluconate Tablets	Oxidation-reduction titration (ceric)
801	Ferrous Sulphate	Oxidation-reduction titration (ceric)
802	Ferrous Sulphate Tablets	Oxidation-reduction titration (ceric)
803	Fexofenadine Capsules	HPLC
804	Fexofenadine Hydrochloride	HPLC
805	Fexofenadine Tablets	HPLC
806	Finasteride	HPLC
807	Finasteride Tablets	HPLC
808	Fingolimod Hydrochloride	HPLC
809	Flavoxate Hydrochloride	Non-Aqueous titration, $HClO_4$
810	Flavoxate Tablets	UV spectroscopy
811	Flucloxacillin Capsules	HPLC
812	Flucloxacillin Oral Solution	HPLC
813	Flucloxacillin Sodium	HPLC
814	Fluconazole	Non-Aqueous titration, $HClO_4$
815	Fluconazole Capsules	HPLC
816	Fluconazole Tablets	HPLC
817	Flucytosine	Non-Aqueous titration, $HClO_4$

Contd...

S. No	Title of Monograph	Assay Method Mentioned
818	Flucytosine Capsules	UV spectroscopy
819	Flucytosine Oral Suspension	HPLC
820	Flucytosine Tablets	UV spectroscopy
821	Fludarabine Phosphate	HPLC
822	Fludarabine Phosphate Injection	HPLC
823	Fludrocortisone Acetate	UV spectroscopy
824	Fludrocortisone Tablets	HPLC
825	Flumazenil	HPLC
826	Flumazenil Injection	HPLC
827	Fluocinolone Acetonide	UV spectroscopy
828	Fluocinolone Cream	HPLC
829	Fluorescein Eye Drops	Gravimetry
830	Fluorescein Injection	HPLC
831	Fluorescein Sodium	Gravimetry
832	Fluorometholone	HPLC
833	Fluorometholone Eye Drops	HPLC
834	Fluorouracil	Non-Aqueous titration, Tetrabutylammonium hydroxide
835	Fluorouracil Injection	UV spectroscopy
836	Fluoxetine Capsules	HPLC
837	Fluoxetine Hydrochloride	HPLC
838	Fluoxetine Oral Solution	HPLC
839	Fluoxetine Tablets	HPLC
840	Flupentixol Decanoate	Non-Aqueous titration, $HClO_4$
841	Flupentixol Injection	HPLC
842	Fluphenazine Decanoate	Non-Aqueous titration, $HClO_4$
843	Fluphenazine Decanoate Injection	Non-Aqueous titration, $HClO_4$
844	Fluphenazine Hydrochloride	Non-Aqueous titration, $HClO_4$
845	Fluphenazine Hydrochloride Injection	UV spectroscopy
846	Fluphenazine Tablets	UV spectroscopy
847	Flurazepam Capsules	UV spectroscopy
848	Flurazepam Hydrochloride	Acid-base titration
849	Flurbiprofen	Acid-base titration

Contd...

S. No	Title of Monograph	Assay Method Mentioned
850	Flurbiprofen Eye Drops	HPLC
851	Flurbiprofen Sodium	HPLC
852	Flurbiprofen Tablets	UV spectroscopy
853	Flutamide	UV spectroscopy
854	Flutamide Capsules	HPLC
855	Flutamide Tablets	HPLC
856	Fluticasone Cream	HPLC
857	Fluticasone Nasal Spray	HPLC
858	Fluticasone Ointment	HPLC
859	Fluticasone Propionate	HPLC
860	Fluticasone Propionate Inhalation	HPLC
861	Fluticasone Propionate Powder for Inhalation	HPLC
862	Fluvastatin Capsules	HPLC
863	Fluvastatin Sodium	Non-Aqueous titration, $HClO_4$
864	Fluvoxamine Maleate	Non-Aqueous titration, $HClO_4$
865	Fluvoxamine Tablets	HPLC
866	Folic Acid	HPLC
867	Folic Acid Tablets	HPLC
868	Fomepizole	HPLC
869	Formoterol Fumarate and Budesonide Powder for Inhalation	HPLC
870	Formoterol Fumarate Dihydrate	Non-Aqueous titration, $HClO_4$
871	Fortified Benzathine Penicillin Injection	For Benzathine Penicillin-Non-aqueous titration, $HClO_4$; For Procaine Penicillin-UV spectroscopy; For Benzylpenicillin sodium-UV spectroscopy
872	Fortified Procaine Penicillin Injection	HPLC
873	Fosinopril Sodium	Acid-base titration
874	Fosinopril Sodium Tablets	HPLC
875	Framycetin Sulphate	Antibiotic assay
876	Frovatriptan Succinate	HPLC

Contd...

S. No	Title of Monograph	Assay Method Mentioned
877	Fructose	No assay mentioned
878	Fructose Injection	Optical rotation
879	Frusemide	Acid-base titration
880	Frusemide Injection	UV spectroscopy
881	Frusemide Tablets	UV spectroscopy
882	Fumaric Acid	Acid-base titration
883	Furazolidone	UV spectroscopy
884	Furazolidone Oral Suspension	UV spectroscopy
885	Furazolidone Tablets	UV spectroscopy
886	Fusidic Acid	Acid-base titration
887	Fusidic Acid Cream	HPLC
888	Galanthamine Hydrobromide	HPLC
889	Gallamine Injection	UV spectroscopy
890	Gallamine Triethiodide	Non-Aqueous titration, $HClO_4$
891	Gefitinib	HPLC
892	Gefitinib Tablets	HPLC
893	Gelatin	No assay mentioned
894	Gemcitabine Hydrochloride	HPLC
895	Gemcitabine Injection	HPLC
896	Gemfibrozil	Acid-base titration
897	Gemfibrozil Capsules	HPLC
898	Gemifloxacin Mesylate	HPLC
899	Gemifloxacin Tablets	HPLC
900	Gentamicin Eye Drops	Antibiotic assay
901	Gentamicin Injection	Antibiotic assay
902	Gentamicin Sulphate	Antibiotic assay
903	Glacial Acetic acid	Acid-base titration
904	Glibenclamide	Acid-base titration
905	Glibenclamide Tablets	HPLC
906	Gliclazide	Non-Aqueous titration, $HClO_4$
907	Gliclazide Tablets	HPLC
908	Glimepiride	HPLC
909	Glimepiride Tablets	HPLC
910	Glipizide	Non-Aqueous titration, (Lithium methoxide)
911	Glipizide Tablets	UV spectroscopy

Contd...

S. No	Title of Monograph	Assay Method Mentioned
912	Glutaraldehyde Solution	Acid-base titration
913	Glycerin	Acid-base titration
914	Glycerin oral solution	Oxidation-reduction titration
915	Glyceryl Monostearate	For monoglycerides - Oxidation-reduction titration (Iodometry); for free glycerin-Oxidation-reduction titration (Iodometry)
916	Glyceryl Trinitrate Tablets	HPLC
917	Glycine	Non-Aqueous titration, $HClO_4$
918	Glycine Irrigation Solution	Acid-base titration
919	Gramicidin	Antibiotic assay
920	Griseofulvin	UV spectroscopy
921	Griseofulvin Tablets	UV spectroscopy
922	Guaiphenesin	Oxidation-Reduction titration (Iodimetry)
923	Half Strength Compound Sodium Lactate and Dextrose Injection	For Sodium-Flame photometry or Atomic Absorption Spectrometry; for Potassium-Flame photometry or Atomic Absorption Spectrometry; for total chlorides-Argentometry (Volhard's method); for calcium chloride-Complexometry titration; for lactate-HPLC; for dextrose-Optical rotation
924	Haloperidol	Non-Aqueous titration, $HClO_4$
925	Haloperidol Injection	UV spectroscopy
926	Haloperidol Oral Solution	UV spectroscopy
927	Haloperidol Tablets	HPLC
928	Hard Gelatin Capsule shells	No assay mentioned
929	Hard Paraffin	No assay mentioned
930	Heavy Kaolin	No assay mentioned
931	Heavy Magnesium Carbonate	Complexometric titration
932	Heavy Magnesium Oxide	Complexometric titration
933	Heparin Injection	Prevention of clotting time of sheep/goat/human plasma
934	Heparin Sodium	Prevention of clotting time of sheep/goat/human plasma

Contd...

S. No	Title of Monograph	Assay Method Mentioned
935	Histamine Phosphate	Non-Aqueous titration, $HClO_4$
936	Histamine Phosphate Injection	Gravimetry
937	Homatropine Eye Drops	HPLC
938	Homatropine Hydrobromide	Non-Aqueous titration, $HClO_4$
939	Homatropine Methylbromide	Argentometry titration
940	Human Insulin	Assay of Insulin
941	Hyaluronidase	Enzyme assay
942	Hyaluronidase Injection	Enzyme assay
943	Hydralazine Hydrochloride	Oxidation-reduction titration (Iodate titration, potentiometry)
944	Hydralazine Injection	Oxidation-reduction titration (Iodate titration, potentiometry)
945	Hydrochloric Acid	Acid-base titration
946	Hydrochlorothiazide	Non-Aqueous titration, Tetrabutylammonium hydroxide
947	Hydrochlorothiazide Tablets	UV spectroscopy
948	Hydrocortisone	UV spectroscopy
949	Hydrocortisone Acetate	UV spectroscopy
950	Hydrocortisone Acetate Injection	HPLC
951	Hydrocortisone Cream	HPLC
952	Hydrocortisone Eye Ointment	HPLC
953	Hydrocortisone Hemisuccinate	UV spectroscopy
954	Hydrocortisone Ointment	HPLC
955	Hydrocortisone Sodium Succinate Injection	UV spectroscopy
956	Hydrogen Peroxide Solution (100 Vol)	Oxidation-reduction titration (Permanganate titration)
957	Hydrogen Peroxide Solution (20 Vol)	Oxidation-reduction titration (Permanganate titration)
958	Hydrogenated Vegetable Oil	No assay mentioned
959	Hydrous Wool Fat	No assay mentioned
960	Hydroxocobalamin	UV spectroscopy
961	Hydroxocobalamin Injection	UV spectroscopy

Contd...

S. No	Title of Monograph	Assay Method Mentioned
962	Hydroxychloroquine Sulphate	Non-Aqueous titration, $HClO_4$
963	Hydroxychloroquine Tablets	HPLC
964	Hydroxyethylcellulose	No assay mentioned
965	Hydroxyprogesterone Hexanoate	UV spectroscopy
966	Hydroxyprogesterone Injection	UV spectroscopy
967	Hydroxypropyl Cellulose	No assay mentioned
968	Hydroxypropyl Methylcellulose Phthalate	No assay mentioned
969	Hydroxypropylmethyl Cellulose	No assay mentioned
970	Hydroxyzine Hydrochloride	Non-Aqueous titration, $HClO_4$
971	Hydroxyzine Oral Solution	HPLC
972	Hydroxyzine Tablets	HPLC
973	Hyoscine Butylbromide	Non-Aqueous titration, $HClO_4$
974	Hyoscine Butylbromide Injection	HPLC
975	Hyoscine Butylbromide Tablets	HPLC
976	Hyoscine Hydrobromide	Non-Aqueous titration, $HClO_4$
977	Hyoscine Hydrobromide Injection	HPLC
978	Hyoscine Hydrobromide Tablets	HPLC
979	Hyoscyamine Injection	HPLC
980	Hyoscyamine Oral Solution	HPLC
981	Hyoscyamine Sulphate	Non-Aqueous titration, $HClO_4$
982	Hyoscyamine Tablets	HPLC
983	Ibudilast	HPLC
984	Ibuprofen	Acid-base titration
985	Ibuprofen Cream	HPLC
986	Ibuprofen Gel	HPLC
987	Ibuprofen Tablets	Acid-base titration
988	Idoxuridine	Non-Aqueous titration, Tetrabutylammonium hydroxide

Contd...

S. No	Title of Monograph	Assay Method Mentioned
989	Idoxuridine Eye Drops	HPLC
990	Ifosafamide Injection (Addendum-2015)	HPLC
991	Ifosfamide (Addendum-2015)	HPLC
992	Ilaprazole	HPLC
993	Iloperidone	Non-Aqueous titration, $HClO_4$
994	Iloperidone Tablets (Addendum-2015)	HPLC
995	Imatinib Capsules	HPLC
996	Imatinib Mesylate	HPLC
997	Imatinib Tablets	HPLC
998	Imidurea	No assay mentioned
999	Imipenem	HPLC
1000	Imipenem and Cilastatin Injection	HPLC
1001	Imipramine Hydrochloride	Non-Aqueous titration, $HClO_4$
1002	Imipramine Tablets	UV spectroscopy
1003	Indapamide	HPLC
1004	Indapamide Tablets	HPLC
1005	Indinavir Capsules	HPLC
1006	Indinavir Sulphate	HPLC
1007	Indomethacin	Acid-base titration
1008	Indomethacin Capsules	UV spectroscopy
1009	Indomethacin Suppositories	UV spectroscopy
1010	Industrial Methylated Spirit	No assay mentioned
1011	Insulin	Assay of Insulin
1012	Insulin Aspart	HPLC
1013	Insulin Aspart Injection	HPLC
1014	Insulin Injection	Assay of Insulin
1015	Insulin Lispro	HPLC
1016	Insulin Lispro Injection	HPLC
1017	Insulin Zinc Suspension	HPLC
1018	Insulin Zinc Suspension (Amorphous)	HPLC
1019	Insulin Zinc Suspension (Crystalline)	HPLC

Contd...

S. No	Title of Monograph	Assay Method Mentioned
1020	Invert Sugar and Sodium Chloride Injection	For Sodium Chloride-Argentometry (Mohr's method); for invert sugar-Gravimetry
1021	Invert Sugar Injection	Gravimetry
1022	Invert Syrup	Oxidation-reduction (reducing sugar, Invert sugar factor method)
1023	Iodine	Oxidation-Reduction titration (Iodimetry)
1024	Iopanoic Acid	Argentometry (potentiometry)
1025	Iopanoic Acid Tablets	Oxidation-reduction titration (Iodate titration)
1026	Ipratropium Bromide	Argentometry (potentiometry)
1027	Ipratropium Inhalation	HPLC
1028	Ipratropium Powder for Inhalation	HPLC
1029	Irbesartan	Non-Aqueous titration, $HClO_4$
1030	Irbesartan and Hydrochlorothiazide Tablets	HPLC
1031	Irbesartan Tablets	Non-Aqueous titration, $HClO_4$
1032	Irinotecan Hydrochloride Trihydrate	HPLC
1033	Irinotecan Injection	HPLC
1034	Iron and Ammonium Citrate	Oxidation-reduction titration (Iodometry)
1035	Iron and Folic Acid Syrup	For Ferrous sulphate-Oxidation-reduction titration (Titanium Chloride); for Folic acid-HPLC
1036	Iron and Folic Acid Tablets	For Ferrous sulphate - Oxidation-reduction titration (ceric ammonium sulphate); for folic acid-HPLC
1037	Iron Dextran Injection	For Iron-Oxidation-reduction titration (Jones reductor, ceric ammonium sulphate)
1038	Isobutane	Gas Chromatography
1039	Isoniazid	HPLC
1040	Isoniazid Tablets	HPLC
1041	Isophane Insulin Injection	Assay of Insulin

Contd...

S. No	Title of Monograph	Assay Method Mentioned
1042	Isoprenaline Hydrochloride	Non-Aqueous titration, $HClO_4$
1043	Isoprenaline Injection	HPLC
1044	Isoprenaline Sulphate	Non-Aqueous titration, $HClO_4$
1045	Isoprenaline Tablets	Visible spectroscopy
1046	Isopropyl Alcohol	No assay mentioned
1047	Isopropyl Myristate	Gas Chromatography
1048	Isopropyl Palmitate	Gas Chromatography
1049	Isopropyl Rubbing Alcohol	Specific gravity
1050	Isosorbide Dinitrate Tablets	HPLC
1051	Isosorbide Mononitrate Tablets	HPLC
1052	Isotretinoin	Non-Aqueous titration, Tetrabutylammonium hydroxide
1053	Isotretinoin Capsules (Addendum-2015)	UV Spectroscopy
1054	Isoxsuprine Hydrochloride	Non-Aqueous titration, $HClO_4$
1055	Isoxsuprine Injection	UV spectroscopy
1056	Isoxsuprine Tablets	UV spectroscopy
1057	Ivermectin	HPLC
1058	Ivermectin Injection	HPLC
1059	Kanamycin Acid Sulphate	Antibiotic assay
1060	Kanamycin Injection	Antibiotic assay
1061	Kanamycin Sulphate	Antibiotic assay
1062	Ketamine Hydrochloride	Non-Aqueous titration, $HClO_4$
1063	Ketamine Injection	UV spectroscopy
1064	Ketoconazole	Non-Aqueous titration, $HClO_4$
1065	Ketoconazole Tablets	HPLC
1066	Ketoprofen	Acid-base titration
1067	Ketoprofen Capsules	UV spectroscopy
1068	Ketorolac Tromethamine	Non-Aqueous titration, $HClO_4$
1069	Ketorolac Tromethamine Injection	HPLC
1070	Ketorolac Tromethamine Tablets	HPLC
1071	Ketotifen Fumarate	Non-Aqueous titration, $HClO_4$

Contd...

S. No	Title of Monograph	Assay Method Mentioned
1072	Ketotifen Fumarate Tablets (Addendum-2015)	UV Spectroscopy
1073	Labetalol Hydrochloride	Non-Aqueous titration, $HClO_4$
1074	Labetalol Injection	UV spectroscopy
1075	Labetalol Tablets	UV spectroscopy
1076	Lacidipine (Addendum-2015)	HPLC
1077	Lacidipine Tablets (Addendum-2015)	HPLC
1078	Lactic Acid	Acid-base titration
1079	Lactose	No assay mentioned
1080	Lactulose	HPLC
1081	Lactulose Oral Powder (Addendum-2015)	HPLC
1082	Lamivudine	HPLC
1083	Lamivudine and Zidovudine Tablets	HPLC
1084	Lamivudine andTenofovir Tablets	HPLC
1085	Lamivudine Oral Solution	HPLC
1086	Lamivudine Tablets	HPLC
1087	Lamivudine, Nevirapine and Stavudine Dispersible Tablets	HPLC
1088	Lamivudine, Nevirapine and Stavudine Tablets	HPLC
1089	Lamivudine, Nevirapine and Zidovudine Paediatric Dispersible Tablets	HPLC
1090	Lamotrigine	HPLC
1091	Lamotrigine Dispersible Tablets	HPLC
1092	Lamotrigine Prolonged-release Tablets	HPLC
1093	Lansoprazole	HPLC
1094	Lansoprazole Gastro-resistant Capsules	HPLC
1095	Lapatinib Ditosylate	HPLC

Contd...

S. No	Title of Monograph	Assay Method Mentioned
1096	Lapatinib Tablets	HPLC
1097	Lecithin	No assay mentioned
1098	Leflunomide	HPLC
1099	Leflunomide Tablets	HPLC
1100	Levamisole Hydrochloride	Acid-base titration
1101	Levamisole Tablets	Non-Aqueous titration, $HClO_4$
1102	Levocetrizine Hydrochloride	Acid-base titration
1103	Levocetrizine Tablets	HPLC
1104	Levodopa	Non-Aqueous titration, $HClO_4$
1105	Levodopa and Carbidopa Tablets	HPLC
1106	Levodopa Capsules	Non-Aqueous titration, $HClO_4$
1107	Levodopa Tablets	Non-Aqueous titration, $HClO_4$
1108	Levodropropizine	Non-Aqueous titration, $HClO_4$
1109	Levofloxacin Hemihydrate	Non-Aqueous titration, $HClO_4$
1110	Levofloxacin Infusion	HPLC
1111	Levofloxacin Injection	HPLC
1112	Levofloxacin Tablets	HPLC
1113	Levonorgestrel	UV spectroscopy
1114	Levonorgestrel and Ethinyloestradiol Tablets	HPLC
1115	Levonorgestrel Tablets	HPLC
1116	Levosalbutamol Hydrochloride	HPLC
1117	Levosalbutamol Inhalation Solution	HPLC
1118	Levosalbutamol Sulphate	HPLC
1119	Light Kaolin	No assay mentioned
1120	Light Liquid Paraffin	No assay mentioned
1121	Light Magnesium Carbonate	Complexometric titration
1122	Light Magnesium Oxide	Complexometric titration
1123	Lignocaine and Adrenaline Injection	For Lignocaine Hydrochloride-Non-Aqueous titration, $HClO_4$; for Adrenaline-HPLC

Contd...

S. No	Title of Monograph	Assay Method Mentioned
1124	Lignocaine and Dextrose Injection	For Lignocaine Hydrochloride-Non-Aqueous titration, $HClO_4$; for dextrose-optical rotation
1125	Lignocaine Gel	Indicator extraction titration
1126	Lignocaine Hydrochloride	Non-Aqueous titration, $HClO_4$
1127	Lignocaine Injection	Non-Aqueous titration, $HClO_4$
1128	Lincomycin Capsules	Gas Chromatography
1129	Lincomycin Hydrochloride	Gas Chromatography
1130	Lindane	Argentometry titration (Volhard method)
1131	Linezolid	HPLC
1132	Linezolid Tablets	HPLC
1133	Liquid Maltitol	HPLC
1134	Liquid Paraffin	No assay mentioned
1135	Liquid Paraffin Emulsion	Gravimetry
1136	Lisinopril	HPLC
1137	Lisinopril Tablets	HPLC
1138	Lithium Carbonate	Acid-base titration
1139	Lithium Carbonate Prolonged-release Tablets	Acid-base titration
1140	Lithium Carbonate Tablets	Acid-base titration
1141	Lomustine	Argentometry (potentiometry)
1142	Lomustine Capsules	UV spectroscopy
1143	Loperamide Capsules	HPLC
1144	Loperamide Hydrochloride	Non-Aqueous titration, $HClO_4$
1145	Loperamide Tablets	HPLC
1146	Lopinavir	HPLC
1147	Lopinavir and Ritonavir Capsules	HPLC
1148	Lopinavir and Ritonavir Tablets	HPLC
1149	Lorazepam	Non-Aqueous titration, Tetrabutylammonium hydroxide
1150	Lorazepam Injection	HPLC
1151	Lorazepam Tablets	UV spectroscopy
1152	Losartan Potassium	HPLC

Contd...

S. No	Title of Monograph	Assay Method Mentioned
1153	Losartan Potassium and Amlodipine Tablets	HPLC
1154	Losartan Potassium and Hydrochlorothiazide Tablets	HPLC
1155	Losartan Tablets	HPLC
1156	Lubiprostone	HPLC
1157	Lynoestrenol	Acid-base titration
1158	Magaldrate	Acid-base titration
1159	Magaldrate Oral Suspension	Acid-base titration
1160	Magaldrate Tablets	Acid-base titration
1161	Magnesium Chloride	Complexometric titration
1162	Magnesium Hydroxide	Complexometric titration
1163	Magnesium Hydroxide Oral Suspension	Acid-base titration
1164	Magnesium Stearate	Complexometric titration
1165	Magnesium Sulphate	Complexometric titration
1166	Magnesium Sulphate Injection	Complexometric titration
1167	Magnesium Trisilicate	For magnesium oxide-Complexometry titration; for silicon dioxide-Gravimetry
1168	Maleic Acid	Acid-base titration
1169	Malic Acid	Acid-base titration
1170	Maltitol	HPLC
1171	Maltodextrin	No assay mentioned
1172	Mannitol	HPLC
1173	Mannitol Injection	Oxidation-Reduction titration (Iodimetry)
1174	Mebendazole	Non-Aqueous titration, $HClO_4$
1175	Mebendazole Tablets	UV spectroscopy
1176	Mebeverine Hydrochloride	Non-Aqueous titration, $HClO_4$
1177	Mebeverine Tablets	UV spectroscopy
1178	Meclizine Hydrochloride	Non-Aqueous titration, $HClO_4$
1179	Meclizine Tablets	Non-Aqueous titration, $HClO_4$
1180	Medroxyprogesterone Acetate	UV spectroscopy

Contd...

S. No	Title of Monograph	Assay Method Mentioned
1181	Medroxyprogesterone Injection	HPLC
1182	Medroxyprogesterone Tablets	HPLC
1183	Mefenamic Acid	Acid-base titration
1184	Mefenamic Acid Capsules	HPLC
1185	Mefloquine Hydrochloride	Non-Aqueous titration, $HClO_4$
1186	Mefloquine Tablets	HPLC
1187	Megestrol Acetate	UV spectroscopy
1188	Megestrol Tablets	UV spectroscopy
1189	Meloxicam	Non-Aqueous titration, $HClO_4$
1190	Meloxicam Oral Suspension	HPLC
1191	Melphalan	Argentometry (potentiometry)
1192	Melphalan Injection	HPLC
1193	Melphalan Tablets	HPLC
1194	Memetasone Aqueous Nasal Spray	HPLC
1195	Menthol	No assay mentioned
1196	Menthol and Benzoin Inhalation	Acid-base titration
1197	Mephentermine Injection	Acid-base titration
1198	Mephentermine Sulphate	Acid-base titration
1199	Mepyramine Maleate	Non-Aqueous titration
1200	Mepyramine Tablets	UV spectroscopy
1201	Mercaptopurine	Non-Aqueous titration, Tetrabutylammonium hydroxide
1202	Mercaptopurine Tablets	UV spectroscopy
1203	Meropenem	HPLC
1204	Meropenem Injection	HPLC
1205	Mesalazine	Acid-base titration
1206	Mesalazine Prolonged-release Tablets	HPLC
1207	Mestranol	Acid-base titration
1208	Metformin Hydrochloride	Non-Aqueous titration, $HClO_4$
1209	Metformin Hydrochloride Prolonged-release Tablets	UV spectroscopy

Contd...

S. No	Title of Monograph	Assay Method Mentioned
1210	Metformin Oral Solution (Addendum-2015)	HPLC
1211	Metformin Tablets	UV spectroscopy
1212	Methadone Hydrochloride	Non-Aqueous titration, $HClO_4$
1213	Methadone Injection	UV spectroscopy
1214	Methadone Linctus	UV spectroscopy
1215	Methadone Oral Solution (Addendum-2015)	HPLC
1216	Methadone Tablets	UV spectroscopy
1217	Methotrexate	HPLC
1218	Methotrexate Injection	HPLC
1219	Methotrexate Tablets	HPLC
1220	Methoxamine Hydrochloride	Non-Aqueous titration, $HClO_4$
1221	Methoxamine Injection	UV spectroscopy
1222	Methyl Salicylate	Acid-base titration
1223	Methyl Salicylate Ointment	Gas Chromatography
1224	Methylcellulose	Oxidation-reduction titration; Methoxyl determination (Iodometry)
1225	Methyldopa	Non-Aqueous titration, $HClO_4$
1226	Methyldopa Tablets	Visible spectroscopy
1227	Methylergometrine Injection	Visible spectroscopy
1228	Methylergometrine Maleate	Visible spectroscopy
1229	Methylergometrine Tablets	Visible spectroscopy
1230	Methylparaben	HPLC
1231	Methylphenidate Hydrochloride (Addendum-2015)	HPLC
1232	Methylphenidate Hydrochloride Prolonged-release Tablets (Addendum-2015)	HPLC
1233	Methylprednisolone	UV spectroscopy
1234	Methylprednisolone Acetate	UV spectroscopy
1235	Methylprednisolone Acetate Injection	HPLC
1236	Methylprednisolone Tablets	HPLC

Contd...

S. No	Title of Monograph	Assay Method Mentioned
1237	Metoclopramide Hydrochloride	Acid-base titration
1238	Metoclopramide Injection	UV spectroscopy
1239	Metoclopramide Syrup	UV spectroscopy
1240	Metoclopramide Tablets	UV spectroscopy
1241	Metolazone (Addendum-2015)	HPLC
1242	Metolazone Tablets (Addendum-2015)	HPLC
1243	Metoprolol Injection	UV spectroscopy
1244	Metoprolol Tablets	UV spectroscopy
1245	Metoprolol Tartrate	Non-Aqueous titration, $HClO_4$
1246	Metronidazole	Non-Aqueous titration, $HClO_4$
1247	Metronidazole Benzoate	Non-Aqueous titration, $HClO_4$
1248	Metronidazole Benzoate Oral Suspension	Non-Aqueous titration, $HClO_4$
1249	Metronidazole Injection	UV spectroscopy
1250	Metronidazole Sterile Suspension	UV spectroscopy
1251	Metronidazole Tablets	Non-Aqueous titration, $HClO_4$
1252	Mexiletine Capsules	UV spectroscopy
1253	Mexiletine Hydrochloride	Non-Aqueous titration, $HClO_4$
1254	Mexiletine Injection	UV spectroscopy
1255	Mianserin Hydrochloride	Acid-base titration
1256	Mianserin Tablets	Gas Chromatography
1257	Miconazole	Non-Aqueous titration, $HClO_4$
1258	Miconazole Cream	Gas Chromatography
1259	Miconazole Nitrate	Non-Aqueous titration, $HClO_4$
1260	Miconazole Pessaries	Gas Chromatography
1261	Microcrystalline Cellulose	Oxidation-reduction titration
1262	Microcrystalline Cellulose and Carboxymethylcellulose Sodium	Non-Aqueous titration, $HClO_4$
1263	Microcrystalline Wax	No assay mentioned
1264	Midazolam	Non-Aqueous titration, $HClO_4$

Contd...

S. No	Title of Monograph	Assay Method Mentioned
1265	Midazolam Injection	HPLC
1266	Midazolam Oral Solution	HPLC
1267	Mifepristone	Non-Aqueous titration, $HClO_4$
1268	Mifepristone Tablets	HPLC
1269	Minoxidil	Non-Aqueous titration, $HClO_4$
1270	Minoxidil Tablets	HPLC
1271	Mirtazapine (Addendum-2015)	Non-Aqueous titration, $HClO_4$
1272	Mirtazapine Tablets (Addendum-2015)	HPLC
1273	Misoprostol	HPLC
1274	Misoprostol Tablets	HPLC
1275	Mitiglinide Calcium Dihydrate	HPLC
1276	Mitomycin	HPLC
1277	Mitomycin Injection	HPLC
1278	Modified Compound Sodium Lactate and Dextrose Injection	For Sodium-Flame photometry or Atomic Absorption Spectrometry; for Potassium-Flame photometry or Atomic Absorption Spectrometry; for total chlorides-Argentometry (Volhard's method); for calcium chloride-Complexometry titration; for lactate-HPLC; for dextrose-Optical rotation
1279	Moexipril Hydrochloride	Non-Aqueous titration, $HClO_4$
1280	Mometasone Cream	HPLC
1281	Mometasone Furoate	UV spectroscopy
1282	Mometasone Ointment	HPLC
1283	Monobasic Sodium Phosphate	Acid-base titration
1284	Monothioglycerol	Oxidation-Reduction titration (Iodimetry)
1285	Montelukast Sodium	HPLC
1286	Montelukast Tablets	HPLC

Contd...

S. No	Title of Monograph	Assay Method Mentioned
1287	Morphine and Atropine Injection	For Atropine Sulphate-Acid-base titration; for morphine sulphate-Acid-base titration
1288	Morphine Injection	HPLC
1289	Morphine Sulphate	Non-Aqueous titration, $HClO_4$
1290	Morphine Tablets	Acid-base titration
1291	Mosapride Citrate Dihydrate	Non-Aqueous titration, $HClO_4$
1292	Mosapride Citrate Tablets	HPLC
1293	Moxifloxacin Eye Drops	HPLC
1294	Moxifloxacin Hydrochloride	HPLC
1295	Multiple Electrolytes and Dextrose Injection Type I	For Sodium-Flame photometry or Atomic absorption spectroscopy; for total potassium-Flame photometry or Atomic absorption spectroscopy; for Magnesium-Complexometry titration; For acetate-HPLC; for total chloride-Argentometry (Volhard method); for dextrose-optical rotation
1296	Multiple Electrolytes and Dextrose Injection Type II	For Sodium-Flame photometry or Atomic absorption spectroscopy; for potassium-Flame photometry or Atomic absorption spectroscopy; for Calcium-Flame photometry or Atomic absorption spectroscopy; for Magnesium-Flame photometry or Atomic absorption spectroscopy; For acetate-HPLC; for total chloride-Argentometry (Volhard method); for dextrose-optical rotation
1297	Multiple Electrolytes and Dextrose Injection Type III	For Sodium-Flame photometry or Atomic absorption spectroscopy; for potassium-Flame photometry or Atomic absorption spectroscopy; For acetate-HPLC; For Phosphate-Visible spectroscopy; for total chloride-Argentometry (Volhard method); for dextrose-optical rotation

Contd...

S. No	Title of Monograph	Assay Method Mentioned
1298	Multiple Electrolytes and Dextrose Injection Type IV	For Sodium-Flame photometry or Atomic absorption spectroscopy; for potassium-Flame photometry or Atomic absorption spectroscopy; For ammonium-Acid-base titration; for total chloride-Argentometry (Volhard method); for dextrose-optical rotation
1299	Multiple Electrolytes and Dextrose Injection Type V	For Sodium-Flame photometry or Atomic absorption spectroscopy; for potassium-Flame photometry or Atomic absorption spectroscopy; for Calcium-Flame photmetry or Atomic absorption spectrometry; for Magnesium-Complexometry titration; for acetate-HPLC; for citrate-HPLC; for total chloride-Argentometry (Volhard method); for dextrose-optical rotation
1300	Multiple Electrolytes Injection Type VI	For total Sodium-Flame photometry or Atomic absorption spectrometry; for Potassium-Flame photometry or Atomic absorption spectrometry; for Calcium-Flame photometry or Atomic absorption spectrometry; for Magnesium-Complexometry titration; for Acetate-HPLC; for Citrate-HPLC; for total Chlorides-Argentometry titration (Volhard method)
1301	Mupirocin	HPLC
1302	Mupirocin Ointment	HPLC
1303	Mustine Hydrochloride	Argentometry titration (Volhard method)
1304	Mustine Injection	Acid-base titration
1305	Mycophenolate Mofetil	Non-Aqueous titration, $HClO_4$
1306	Mycophenolate Mofetil Capsules	HPLC
1307	Myristic Acid	Gas Chromatography

Contd...

S. No	Title of Monograph	Assay Method Mentioned
1308	Nabumetone (Addendum-2015)	HPLC
1309	Nabumetone Tablets (Addendum-2015)	HPLC
1310	Nalidixic Acid	Acid-base titration
1311	Nalidixic Acid Tablets	UV spectroscopy
1312	Nalorphine Hydrochloride	UV spectroscopy
1313	Nalorphine Injection	UV spectroscopy
1314	Naloxone Hydrochloride	Acid-base titration
1315	Naloxone Injection	HPLC
1316	Naltrexone Hydrochloride	Acid-base titration
1317	Naltrexone Tablets	HPLC
1318	Nandrolone Decanoate	UV spectroscopy
1319	Nandrolone Decanoate Injection	UV spectroscopy
1320	Nandrolone Phenylpropionate	UV spectroscopy
1321	Nandrolone Phenylpropionate Injection	UV spectroscopy
1322	Naphazoline Nitrate	Non-Aqueous titration, $HClO_4$
1323	Naproxcinod	HPLC
1324	Naproxen	Acid-base titration
1325	Naproxen Oral Suspension	UV spectroscopy
1326	Naproxen Prolonged-release Tablets	HPLC
1327	Naproxen Suppositories	HPLC
1328	Naproxen Tablets	UV spectroscopy
1329	Natamycin	HPLC
1330	Natamycin Ophthalmic Suspension	HPLC
1331	Nebivolol Hydrochloride	HPLC
1332	Nebivolol Tablets	HPLC
1333	Nelfinariv Mesylate Oral Powder	HPLC
1334	Nelfinavir Mesylate	HPLC
1335	Nelfinavir Tablets	HPLC
1336	Neomycin Eye Drops	Antibiotic assay
1337	Neomycin Eye Ointment	Antibiotic assay

Contd...

S. No	Title of Monograph	Assay Method Mentioned
1338	Neomycin Sulphate	Antibiotic assay
1339	Neostigmine Bromide	Non-Aqueous titration, $HClO_4$
1340	Neostigmine Injection	UV spectroscopy
1341	Neostigmine Methylsulphate	Acid-base titration
1342	Neostigmine Tablets	Acid-base titration
1343	Neotame	HPLC
1344	Netilmicin Injection (Addendum-2015)	HPLC
1345	Netilmicin Sulphate	Antibiotic assay
1346	Nevirapine	HPLC
1347	Nevirapine Oral Suspension	HPLC
1348	Nevirapine Tablets	HPLC
1349	Niclosamide	Non-Aqueous titration, Tetrabutylammonium hydroxide
1350	Niclosamide Tablets	Non-Aqueous titration, Tetrabutylammonium hydroxide
1351	Nicorandil	HPLC
1352	Nicorandil Prolonged-release Tablets	HPLC
1353	Nicorandil Tablets	HPLC
1354	Nicotinamide	Non-Aqueous titration, $HClO_4$
1355	Nicotinamide Tablets	UV spectroscopy
1356	Nicotinic Acid	Acid-base titration
1357	Nicotinic Acid Tablets	Acid-base titration
1358	Nicoumalone	Acid-base titration
1359	Nicoumalone Tablets	UV spectroscopy
1360	Nifedipine	Oxidation-reduction titration (ceric)
1361	Nifedipine Capsules	UV spectroscopy
1362	Nifedipine Prolonged-release Tablets	UV spectroscopy
1363	Nifedipine Tablets	UV spectroscopy
1364	Nikethamide	Non-Aqueous titration, $HClO_4$
1365	Nikethamide Injection	UV spectroscopy
1366	Nitrazepam	Non-Aqueous titration, $HClO_4$
1367	Nitrazepam Tablets	UV spectroscopy
1368	Nitrofurantoin	UV spectroscopy

Contd...

S. No	Title of Monograph	Assay Method Mentioned
1369	Nitrofurantoin Tablets	UV spectroscopy
1370	Nitrofurazone	UV spectroscopy
1371	Nitrous Oxide	Gasometry
1372	Noradrenaline Bitartrate	Non-Aqueous titration, $HClO_4$
1373	Noradrenaline Bitartrate Injection	UV spectroscopy
1374	Norethisterone	Acid-base titration
1375	Norethisterone Tablets	HPLC
1376	Norfloxacin	Non-Aqueous titration, $HClO_4$
1377	Norfloxacin Eye Drops	HPLC
1378	Norfloxacin Tablets	HPLC
1379	Norgestrel	UV spectroscopy
1380	Norgestrel and Ethinyloestradiol Tablets	HPLC
1381	Nortriptyline Hydrochloride	Non-Aqueous titration, $HClO_4$
1382	Nortriptyline Tablets	HPLC
1383	Noscapine	Non-Aqueous titration, $HClO_4$
1384	Noscapine Linctus	UV spectroscopy
1385	Novabiocin Sodium	Antibiotic assay
1386	Nystatin	Antibiotic assay
1387	Nystatin Ointment	Antibiotic assay
1388	Nystatin Pessaries	Antibiotic assay
1389	Nystatin Tablets	Antibiotic assay
1390	Octyldodecanol	Gas Chromatography
1391	Oestradiol Benzoate	UV spectroscopy
1392	Oestradiol Injection	HPLC
1393	Ofloxacin	Non-Aqueous titration, $HClO_4$
1394	Ofloxacin Infusion	HPLC
1395	Ofloxacin Ophthalmic Solution	HPLC
1396	Ofloxacin Oral Suspension	HPLC
1397	Ofloxacin Tablets	HPLC
1398	Olanzapine	Non-Aqueous titration, $HClO_4$
1399	Olanzapine Tablets	HPLC
1400	Oleic Acid	No assay mentioned
1401	Omeprazole	HPLC

Contd....

S. No	Title of Monograph	Assay Method Mentioned
1402	Omeprazole Gastro-resistant Capsules	HPLC
1403	Ondansetron	HPLC
1404	Ondansetron Hydrochloride	HPLC
1405	Ondansetron Injection	HPLC
1406	Ondansetron Oral Solution	HPLC
1407	Ondansetron Orally Disintegration Tablets	HPLC
1408	Ondansetron Tablets	HPLC
1409	Oral Rehydration Salts	For sodium- Flame photometry or Atomic absorption spectrophotometry ; for potassium- Flame photometry or Atomic absorption spectrophotometry; for total chlorides- Argentometry (Mohr's method); for citrate-Non-Aqueous titration, $HClO_4$; for dextrose-optical rotation
1410	Ormeloxifene Hydrochloride	HPLC
1411	Ormeloxifene Hydrochloride Tablets	HPLC
1412	Ornidazole	Non-Aqueous titration, $HClO_4$
1413	Ornidazole Injection	HPLC
1414	Ornidazole Tablets	Non-Aqueous titration, $HClO_4$
1415	Orphenadrine Citrate	Non-Aqueous titration, $HClO_4$
1416	Orphenadrine Hydrochloride	Non-Aqueous titration, $HClO_4$
1417	Orphenadrine Tablets	Non-Aqueous titration, $HClO_4$
1418	Oseltamivir Capsules	HPLC
1419	Oseltamivir Oral Suspension	HPLC
1420	Oseltamivir Phosphate	HPLC
1421	Oxacillin Capsules	HPLC
1422	Oxacillin Sodium	HPLC
1423	Oxazepam	Non-Aqueous titration, $HClO_4$
1424	Oxazepam Tablets	UV spectroscopy
1425	Oxcarbazepine	HPLC
1426	Oxcarbazepine Tablets	HPLC
1427	Oxprenolol Hydrochloride	Non-Aqueous titration, $HClO_4$
1428	Oxprenolol Tablets	UV spectroscopy

Contd...

S. No	Title of Monograph	Assay Method Mentioned
1429	Oxygen	Gasometry
1430	Oxygen 93 Percent	Gasometry
1431	Oxytetracycline Capsules	Antibiotic assay
1432	Oxytetracycline Dihydrate	Antibiotic assay
1433	Oxytetracycline Eye Ointment	Antibiotic assay
1434	Oxytetracycline Hydrochloride	Antibiotic assay
1435	Oxytetracycline Hydrochloride Injection	Antibiotic assay
1436	Oxytetracycline Injection	Antibiotic assay
1437	Oxytocin	HPLC
1438	Oxytocin Injection	HPLC
1439	Oxytocin Nasal Solution	HPLC
1440	Ozagrel Hydrochloride	HPLC
1441	Paclitaxel	HPLC
1442	Paclitaxel Injection	HPLC
1443	Pancreatin	For Protease activity-Acid-base titration (enzyme activity); for lipase activity-Acid-base (enzyme activity); for amylase acitivity-enzyme activity
1444	Pantoprazole Gastro-resistant Tablets	HPLC
1445	Pantoprazole Sodium	HPLC
1446	Paracetamol	Oxidation-reduction titration (ceric)
1447	Paracetamol Infusion	HPLC
1448	Paracetamol Oral Suspension	HPLC
1449	Paracetamol Paediatric Oral Suspension	HPLC
1450	Paracetamol Syrup	HPLC
1451	Paracetamol Tablets	UV spectroscopy
1452	Paraffin Ointment	No assay mentioned
1453	Paraldehyde	No assay mentioned
1454	Parecoxib Sodium	Non-Aqueous titration, $HClO_4$
1455	Paroxetine Hydrochloride	HPLC
1456	Paroxetine Tablets	HPLC

Contd...

S. No	Title of Monograph	Assay Method Mentioned
1457	Pemetrexed Disodium	HPLC
1458	Penicillamine	Non-Aqueous titration, $HClO_4$
1459	Penicillamine Tablets	Complexometric titration (Mercuric nitrate titration)
1460	Pentaerythritol Tetranitrate Tablets	Visible spectroscopy
1461	Pentamidine Injection	Non-Aqueous titration, Tetrabutylammonium hydroxide
1462	Pentamidine Isethionate	Non-Aqueous titration, Tetrabutylammonium hydroxide
1463	Pentazocine	Non-Aqueous titration, $HClO_4$
1464	Pentazocine Hydrochloride	Non-Aqueous titration, $HClO_4$
1465	Pentazocine Injection	UV spectroscopy
1466	Pentazocine Lactate	Non-Aqueous titration, Tetrabutylammonium hydroxide
1467	Pentazocine Tablets	UV spectroscopy
1468	Pentobarbitone Sodium	Acid-base titration
1469	Pentobarbitone Tablets	Gravimetry
1470	Pepsin	Egg albumin assay
1471	Peritoneal Dialysis Solution	For sodium- Flame photometry or Atomic absorption spectrophotometry ; for potassium- Flame photometry or Atomic absorption spectrophotometry; for calcium- Flame photometry or Atomic absorption spectrophotometry; for magnesium-Complexometry titration; for total chlorides- Argentometry (Volhard method); for acetate-HPLC; for lactate- HPLC; for sodium bicarbonate- Acid-base titration; for lactate and bicarbonate-HPLC; for dextrose- Oxidation-reduction titration (Iodometry)
1472	Perphenazine	Non-Aqueous titration, $HClO_4$
1473	Perphenazine Tablets	UV spectroscopy
1474	Pethidine Hydrochloride	Non-Aqueous titration, $HClO_4$
1475	Pethidine Injection	HPLC

Contd...

S. No	Title of Monograph	Assay Method Mentioned
1476	Pethidine Tablets	Non-Aqueous titration, $HClO_4$
1477	Petrolatum	No assay mentioned
1478	Phenindione	Oxidation-reduction titration (Iodometry)
1479	Phenindione Tablets	UV spectroscopy
1480	Pheniramine Injection	UV spectroscopy
1481	Pheniramine Maleate	Non-Aqueous titration, $HClO_4$
1482	Pheniramine Tablets	UV spectroscopy
1483	Phenobarbitone	Acid-base titration
1484	Phenobarbitone Injection	Argentometry titration
1485	Phenobarbitone Sodium	Acid-base titration
1486	Phenobarbitone Sodium Tablets	Gravimetry
1487	Phenobarbitone Tablets	Gravimetry
1488	Phenol	Oxidation-reduction titration (Iodometry)
1489	Phenolphthalein	Oxidation-Reduction titration (Iodimetry)
1490	Phenoxyethanol	Acid-base titration
1491	Phenoxymethylpenicillin Potassium	HPLC
1492	Phenoxymethylpenicillin Potassium Tablets	HPLC
1493	Phentolamine Injection	UV spectroscopy
1494	Phentolamine Mesylate	Non-Aqueous titration, Tetrabutylammonium hydroxide
1495	Phenylephrine Hydrochoride	Acid-base titration
1496	Phenylephrine Injection	UV spectroscopy
1497	Phenylethyl Alcohol	No assay mentioned
1498	Phenylmercuric Acetate	Precipitation titration (Ammonium thiocyanate)
1499	Phenylmercuric Nitrate	Precipitation titration (Ammonium thiocyanate)
1500	Phenyramidol Hydrochloride	Non-Aqueous titration, $HClO_4$
1501	Phenyramidol Tablets	HPLC
1502	Phenytoin	Non-Aqueous titration, (Sodium methoxide)

Contd...

S. No	Title of Monograph	Assay Method Mentioned
1503	Phenytoin Capsules	Non-Aqueous titration, Tetrabutylammonium hydroxide
1504	Phenytoin Injection	Acid-base titration
1505	Phenytoin Oral Suspension	Gravimetry
1506	Phenytoin Sodium	Acid-base titration
1507	Phenytoin Tablets	Non-Aqueous titration, Tetrabutylammonium hydroxide
1508	Pholcodine	Non-Aqueous titration, $HClO_4$
1509	Pholcodine Linctus	Non-Aqueous titration, $HClO_4$
1510	Phosphoric Acid	Acid-base titration
1511	Physostigmine Injection	Non-Aqueous titration, $HClO_4$
1512	Physostigmine Salicylate	Non-Aqueous titration, $HClO_4$
1513	Pilocarpine Eye Drops	HPLC
1514	Pilocarpine Nitrate	Non-Aqueous titration, $HClO_4$
1515	Pimozide	Non-Aqueous titration, $HClO_4$
1516	Pimozide Tablets	HPLC
1517	Pindolol	Acid-base titration
1518	Pindolol Tablets	UV spectroscopy
1519	Pioglitazone Hydrochloride	HPLC
1520	Pioglitazone Tablets	HPLC
1521	Piperacillin	HPLC
1522	Piperacillin Intravenous Infusion	HPLC
1523	Piperazine Adipate	Non-Aqueous titration, $HClO_4$
1524	Piperazine Adipate Tablets	Gravimetry
1525	Piperazine Citrate	Non-Aqueous titration, $HClO_4$
1526	Piperazine Citrate Syrup	Gravimetry
1527	Piperazine Hydrate	Non-Aqueous titration, $HClO_4$
1528	Piperazine Phosphate	Gravimetry
1529	Piperazine Phosphate Tablets	Gravimetry
1530	Piracetam	HPLC
1531	Piroxicam	HPLC
1532	Piroxicam Capsules	HPLC
1533	Pitavastatin Calcium	HPLC
1534	Plaster of Paris	No assay mentioned
1535	Polacrilin Potassium	No assay mentioned

Contd...

S. No	Title of Monograph	Assay Method Mentioned
1536	Poloxamers	No assay mentioned
1537	Polyethylene Glycol 1500	No assay mentioned
1538	Polyethylene Glycol 4000	No assay mentioned
1539	Polyethylene Glycol 6000	No assay mentioned
1540	Polyoxyl 35 Castor Oil	No assay mentioned
1541	Polyoxyl 40 Hydrogenated Castor Oil	No assay mentioned
1542	Polysorbate 20	No assay mentioned
1543	Polysorbate 80	No assay mentioned
1544	Polyvinyl Acetate Phthalate	UV spectroscopy
1545	Polyvinyl Alcohol	No assay mentioned
1546	Potassium Chloride	Argentometry titration (Mohr's method)
1547	Potassium Chloride for Dextrose Injection	For potassium chloride-Argentometry (Mohr's method); for dextrose-optical rotation
1548	Potassium Chloride for Injection	For potassium-Atomic absorption spectrometry
1549	Potassium Chloride, Sodium Chloride and Dextrose Injection	For Sodium-Flame photometry or Atomic absorption spectrophotometry; for potassium-Flame photometry or Atomic absorption spectrophotometry; for total chloride-Argentometry (Volhard's Method); for dextrose-optical rotation
1550	Potassium Citrate	Non-Aqueous titration, $HClO_4$
1551	Potassium Clavulanate	HPLC
1552	Potassium Clavulanate Diluted	HPLC
1553	Potassium Iodide	Indicator extraction titration
1554	Potassium Permanganate	Oxidation-reduction titration (Iodometry)
1555	Potassium Sorbate	Non-Aqueous titration, $HClO_4$
1556	Povidone	No assay mentioned
1557	Povidone-Iodine	Oxidation-reduction titration
1558	Povidone-Iodine Solution	Oxidation-reduction titration
1559	Pralidoxime Chloride	UV spectroscopy

Contd...

S. No	Title of Monograph	Assay Method Mentioned
1560	Pralidoxime Chloride Injection	UV spectroscopy
1561	Pravastatin Sodium	HPLC
1562	Pravastatin Tablets	HPLC
1563	Praziquantel	HPLC
1564	Praziquantel Tablets	HPLC
1565	Prazosin Hydrochloride	Non-Aqueous titration, $HClO_4$
1566	Prazosin Tablets	HPLC
1567	Prednisolone	UV spectroscopy
1568	Prednisolone Acetate	UV spectroscopy
1569	Prednisolone Sodium Phosphate	UV spectroscopy
1570	Prednisolone Sodium Phosphate Eye Drops	HPLC
1571	Prednisolone Sodium Phosphate Injection	HPLC
1572	Prednisolone Tablets	HPLC
1573	Prednisone	UV spectroscopy
1574	Prednisone Tablets	HPLC
1575	Pregabalin	HPLC
1576	Pregabalin Capsules	HPLC
1577	Pregalatinised Starch	No assay mentioned
1578	Primaquine Phosphate	Non-Aqueous titration, $HClO_4$
1579	Primaquine Tablets	HPLC
1580	Probenecid	Acid-base titration
1581	Probenecid Tablets	UV spectroscopy
1582	Procainamide Hydrochloride	Diazotisation titration (Nitrite titration)
1583	Procainamide Injection	Diazotisation titration (Nitrite titration)
1584	Procainamide Tablets	Diazotisation titration (Nitrite titration)
1585	Procaine and Adrenaline Injection	For procaine hydrochloride-Acid-base titration; for Adrenaline-Visible spectroscopy
1586	Procaine Hydrochloride	Diazotisation titration (Nitrite titration)

Contd...

S. No	Title of Monograph	Assay Method Mentioned
1587	Procaine Penicillin	For benzyl penicillin and procaine-HPLC
1588	Procarbazine Hydrochloride	Acid-base titration
1589	Prochlorperazine Injection	UV spectroscopy
1590	Prochlorperazine Maleate	Non-Aqueous titration, $HClO_4$
1591	Prochlorperazine Mesylate	Non-Aqueous titration, $HClO_4$
1592	Prochlorperazine Tablets	UV spectroscopy
1593	Procyclidine Hydrochloride	Non-Aqueous titration, $HClO_4$
1594	Procyclidine Tablets	Visible spectroscopy
1595	Progesterone	UV spectroscopy
1596	Progesterone Injectable Suspension	HPLC
1597	Progesterone Injection	UV spectroscopy
1598	Proguanil Hydrochloride	Non-Aqueous titration, $HClO_4$
1599	Proguanil Tablets	Visible spectroscopy
1600	Promazine Hydrochloride	Acid-base titration
1601	Promazine Tablets	UV spectroscopy
1602	Promethazine Hydrochloride	Acid-base titration
1603	Promethazine Injection	UV spectroscopy
1604	Promethazine Syrup	UV spectroscopy
1605	Promethazine Tablets	UV spectroscopy
1606	Promethazine Theoclate	Non-Aqueous titration, $HClO_4$
1607	Promethazine Theoclate Tablets	UV spectroscopy
1608	Propane	Gas Chromatography
1609	Propionic Acid	Acid-base titration
1610	Propofol	HPLC
1611	Propofol Injection	HPLC
1612	Propranolol Hydrochloride	Acid-base titration
1613	Propranolol Injection	UV spectroscopy
1614	Propranolol Tablets	UV spectroscopy
1615	Propyl Gallate	No assay mentioned
1616	Propylene Glycol	No assay mentioned
1617	Propyliodone	Oxidation-reduction titration (Iodometry)

Contd...

S. No	Title of Monograph	Assay Method Mentioned
1618	Propyliodone Injectable Oil Suspension	Oxidation-reduction titration (Iodometry)
1619	Propylparaben	HPLC
1620	Propylthiouracil	Acid-base titration
1621	Propylthiouracil Tablets	Mercurimetric titration
1622	Propyphenazone	Non-Aqueous titration, $HClO_4$
1623	Protamine Sulphate	Visible spectroscopy
1624	Protamine Sulphate Injection	Visible spectroscopy
1625	Prothionamide	HPLC
1626	Prothionamide Tablets	HPLC
1627	Protriptyline Hydrochloride	Non-Aqueous titration, $HClO_4$
1628	Protriptyline Tablets	UV spectroscopy
1629	Pseudoephedrine Hydrochloride	Non-Aqueous titration, $HClO_4$
1630	Pseudoephedrine Syrup	HPLC
1631	Pseudoephedrine Tablets	HPLC
1632	Psoralen	UV spectroscopy
1633	Purified Rayon	No assay mentioned
1634	Purified Water	No assay mentioned
1635	Pyantel Pamoate Oral Suspension	HPLC
1636	Pyrantel Pamoate	Non-Aqueous titration, $HClO_4$
1637	Pyrazinamide	Acid-base titration
1638	Pyrazinamide Tablets	UV spectroscopy
1639	Pyridostigmine Bromide	Non-Aqueous titration, $HClO_4$
1640	Pyridostigmine Injection	UV spectroscopy
1641	Pyridostigmine Tablets	UV spectroscopy
1642	Pyridoxine Hydrochloride	Non-Aqueous titration, $HClO_4$
1643	Pyridoxine Tablets	UV spectroscopy
1644	Pyrimethamine	Non-Aqueous titration, $HClO_4$
1645	Pyrimethamine and sulphadoxine Tablets	HPLC
1646	Pyrimethamine Tablets	UV spectroscopy
1647	Quetiapine Fumarate	HPLC
1648	Quetiapine Tablets	HPLC
1649	Quinalbarbitone Sodium	Acid-base titration

Contd...

S. No	Title of Monograph	Assay Method Mentioned
1650	Quinalbarbitone Tablets	Gravimetry
1651	Quinidine Sulphate	Non-Aqueous titration, $HClO_4$
1652	Quinidine Tablets	Non-Aqueous titration, $HClO_4$
1653	Quinine Bisulphate	Non-Aqueous titration, $HClO_4$
1654	Quinine Bisulphate Tablets	Non-Aqueous titration, $HClO_4$
1655	Quinine Dihydrochloride	Non-Aqueous titration, $HClO_4$
1656	Quinine Dihydrochloride Injection	Non-Aqueous titration, $HClO_4$
1657	Quinine Sulphate	Non-Aqueous titration, $HClO_4$
1658	Quinine Tablets	Non-Aqueous titration, $HClO_4$
1659	Quiniodochlor	Non-Aqueous titration, Tetrabutylammonium hydroxide
1660	Quiniodochlor and Hydrocortisone Cream	For hydrocortisone-HPLC; for quiniodochlor-Visible spectroscopy
1661	Quiniodochlor and Hydrocortisone Ointment	For hydrocortisone-HPLC; for quiniodochlor-Visible spectroscopy
1662	Quiniodochlor Cream	Gas Chromatography
1663	Quiniodochlor Ointment	Gas Chromatography
1664	Quiniodochlor Tablets	Visible spectroscopy
1665	Rabeprazole Gastro-resistant Tablets	HPLC
1666	Rabeprazole Injection (Addendum-2015)	HPLC
1667	Rabeprazole Sodium	HPLC
1668	Racecadotril	HPLC
1669	Racecadotril Capsules	HPLC
1670	Racecadotril Sachet	HPLC
1671	Raloxifene Hydrochloride	HPLC
1672	Raloxifene Hydrochloride Tablets (Addendum-2015)	HPLC
1673	Ramelteon	HPLC
1674	Ramipril	Acid-base titration
1675	Ramipril and Hydrochlorothiazide Tablets	HPLC
1676	Ramipril Capsules	HPLC

Contd...

S. No	Title of Monograph	Assay Method Mentioned
1677	Ramipril Tablets	HPLC
1678	Ranitidine Hydrochloride	HPLC
1679	Ranitidine Injection	HPLC
1680	Ranitidine Oral Solution (Addendum-2015)	HPLC
1681	Ranitidine Tablets	HPLC
1682	Rebamipide	HPLC
1683	Reboxetine Methanesulphonate	HPLC
1684	Repaglinide	Non-Aqueous titration, $HClO_4$
1685	Repaglinide Tablets	HPLC
1686	Reserpine	For total alkaloids-Non-Aqueous titration, $HClO_4$; for reserpine-UV spectroscopy
1687	Reserpine Injection	UV spectroscopy
1688	Reserpine Tablets	UV spectroscopy
1689	Ribavirin	HPLC
1690	Ribavirin Inhalation Solution	HPLC
1691	Riboflavin	Visible spectroscopy
1692	Riboflavin Sodium Phosphate	Visible spectroscopy
1693	Riboflavin Tablets	Visible spectroscopy
1694	Rifampicin	HPLC
1695	Rifampicin and Isoniazid Tablets	HPLC
1696	Rifampicin Capsules	HPLC
1697	Rifampicin Oral Suspension	HPLC
1698	Rifampicin Tablets	HPLC
1699	Rifampicin, Isoniazid and Ethambutol Tablets	For Rifampicin and isoniazid-HPLC; for ethambutol hydrochloride-HPLC
1700	Rifampicin, Isoniazid and Pyrazinamide Tablets	For Rifampicin and isoniazid and pyrazinamide-HPLC
1701	Rifampicin, Isoniazid, Pyrazinamide and Ethambutol Tablets	For Rifampicin and isoniazid and pyrazinamide-HPLC
1702	Rilpivirine	HPLC
1703	Risedronate Sodium	HPLC

Contd...

S. No	Title of Monograph	Assay Method Mentioned
1704	Ritodrine Hydrochloride	HPLC
1705	Ritodrine Injection	HPLC
1706	Ritodrine Tablets	HPLC
1707	Ritonavir	HPLC
1708	Ritonavir Capsules	HPLC
1709	Ritonavir Tablets	HPLC
1710	Rizatriptan Benzoate	HPLC
1711	Rizatriptan Tablets	HPLC
1712	Roflumilast	HPLC
1713	Rosuvastatin Calcium	HPLC
1714	Rosuvastatin Tablets	HPLC
1715	Roxithromycin	HPLC
1716	Roxithromycin Tablets	HPLC
1717	Rufinamide	HPLC
1718	Rupatadine Fumarate	HPLC
1719	Saccharin	Acid-base titration
1720	Saccharin Sodium	Non-Aqueous titration, $HClO_4$
1721	Safinamide Methane Sulphonate	HPLC
1722	Salbutamol	Non-Aqueous titration, $HClO_4$
1723	Salbutamol Inhalation	Visible spectroscopy
1724	Salbutamol Injection	Visible spectroscopy
1725	Salbutamol Sulphate	Non-Aqueous titration, $HClO_4$
1726	Salbutamol Syrup	Visible spectroscopy
1727	Salbutamol Tablets	HPLC
1728	Salicylic Acid	Acid-base titration
1729	Salicylic Acid Ointment	Acid-base titration
1730	Salmeterol and Fluticasone Propionate Inhalation	HPLC
1731	Salmeterol and Fluticasone Propionate Powder for Inhalation	HPLC
1732	Salmeterol Xinafoate	HPLC
1733	S-Amlodipine besylate	HPLC
1734	S-Amlodipine besylate tablets	HPLC

Contd...

S. No	Title of Monograph	Assay Method Mentioned
1735	Saquinavir	HPLC
1736	Saquinavir Capsules	HPLC
1737	Saquinavir Mesylate	HPLC
1738	Saquinavir Mesylate Tablets	HPLC
1739	Secnidazole	HPLC
1740	Secnidazole Tablets	HPLC
1741	Selegiline Hydrochloride	Non-Aqueous titration, $HClO_4$
1742	Selegiline Tablets	HPLC
1743	Seratrodast	HPLC
1744	Serratiopeptidase	Enzyme assay
1745	Serratiopeptidase Tablets	Enzyme assay
1746	Sertraline Hydrochloride	HPLC
1747	Sertraline Tablets	HPLC
1748	Sildenafil Citrate	HPLC
1749	Sildenafil Tablets	HPLC
1750	Silver Nitrate	Argentometry titration (Volhard method)
1751	Silver Sulphadiazine	HPLC
1752	Silver Sulphadiazine Cream	HPLC
1753	Simvastatin	HPLC
1754	Simvastatin Tablets	HPLC
1755	Sisomicin Sulphate	Antibiotic assay
1756	Sisomicin Sulphate Injection	Antibiotic assay
1757	Sitagliptin Phosphate (Addendum-2015)	HPLC
1758	Sitagliptin Tablets (Addendum-2015)	HPLC
1759	Sodium Acetate	Non-Aqueous titration, $HClO_4$
1760	Sodium Alginate	No assay mentioned
1761	Sodium Aminosalicylate	HPLC
1762	Sodium Aminosalicylate Tablets	HPLC
1763	Sodium Ascorbate	Oxidation-Reduction titration (Iodimetry)
1764	Sodium Benzoate	Non-Aqueous titration, $HClO_4$
1765	Sodium Bicarbonate	Acid-base titration

Contd...

S. No	Title of Monograph	Assay Method Mentioned
1766	Sodium Bicarbonate Injection	Acid-base titration
1767	Sodium Carbonate	Acid-base titration
1768	Sodium Chloride	Argentometry titration (Volhard method)
1769	Sodium Chloride and Dextrose Injection	For Sodium chloride-Argentometry (Mohr's method); for dextrose-Optical rotation
1770	Sodium Chloride and Fructose Injection	For Sodium Chloride-Argentometry (Mohr's method); for Fructose-Optical rotation
1771	Sodium Chloride Hypertonic Injection	Argentometry titration (Volhard method)
1772	Sodium Chloride Injection	Argentometry titration (Volhard method)
1773	Sodium Chloride Irrigation Solution	Argentometry titration (Mohr's method)
1774	Sodium Citrate	Non-Aqueous titration, $HClO_4$
1775	Sodium Citrate Eye drops	Non-Aqueous titration, $HClO_4$
1776	Sodium Citrate Irrigation Solution	Non-Aqueous titration, $HClO_4$
1777	Sodium Diatrizoate	Oxidation-reduction titration (Iodate titration-Iodometry)
1778	Sodium Diatrizoate Injection	Oxidation-reduction titration (Iodate titration-Iodometry)
1779	Sodium Dihydrogen Phosphate Dihydrate	Acid-base titration
1780	Sodium Fluoride	Non-Aqueous titration, $HClO_4$
1781	Sodium Formaldehyde Sulphoxylate	Oxidation-Reduction titration (Iodimetry)
1782	Sodium Fusidate	Acid-base titration
1783	Sodium Hydroxide	Acid-base titration
1784	Sodium Lactate Injection	Acid-base titration
1785	Sodium Lauryl Sulphate	Indicator extraction titration
1786	Sodium Metabisulphite	Oxidation-Reduction titration (Iodimetry)
1787	Sodium Methylparaben	HPLC
1788	Sodium Nitrite (Addendum-2015)	Oxidation-reduction titration (Iodometry)

Contd...

S. No	Title of Monograph	Assay Method Mentioned
1789	Sodium Nitrite Injection (Addendum-2015)	Oxidation-reduction titration (Iodometry)
1790	Sodium Nitroprusside	Argentometry titration
1791	Sodium Nitroprusside Injection	HPLC
1792	Sodium Phosphate	Acid-base titration
1793	Sodium Propylparaben	HPLC
1794	Sodium Salicylate	Non-Aqueous titration, $HClO_4$
1795	Sodium Starch Glycollate	Non-Aqueous titration, $HClO_4$
1796	Sodium Stibogluconate	Oxidation-reduction titration (Ferric ammonium sulphate)
1797	Sodium Stibogluconate injection	Oxidation-reduction titration (Ferric ammonium sulphate)
1798	Sodium Thiosulphate	Oxidation-Reduction titration (Iodimetry)
1799	Sodium Thiosulphate Injection	Oxidation-Reduction titration (Iodimetry)
1800	Sodium Valproate	Non-Aqueous titration, $HClO_4$
1801	Sodium Valproate Gastro-resistant Tablets	Gas Chromatography
1802	Sodium Valproate Injection	Gas Chromatography
1803	Sodium Valproate Oral Solution	Acid-base titration
1804	Sodium Valproate Tablets	Acid-base titration
1805	Soluble aspirin tablets	Oxidation-reduction titration (Iodometry)
1806	Sorafenib Tablets	HPLC
1807	Sorafenib Tosylate	HPLC
1808	Sorbic Acid	Acid-base titration
1809	Sorbitan Oleate	No assay mentioned
1810	Sorbitol	HPLC
1811	Sorbitol Solution (70 percent) (Crystallising)	HPLC
1812	Sorbitol Solution (70 percent) (Non-Crystallising)	HPLC
1813	Soyabean Oil	No assay mentioned
1814	Spironolactone	UV spectroscopy

Contd...

S. No	Title of Monograph	Assay Method Mentioned
1815	Spironolactone Tablets	UV spectroscopy
1816	Stavudine	HPLC
1817	Stavudine and Lamivudine Tablets	HPLC
1818	Stavudine Capsules	HPLC
1819	Stavudine Oral Solution	HPLC
1820	Stearic Acid	Gas Chromatography
1821	Stearyl Alcohol	Gas Chromatography
1822	Sterile Water for Inhalation (Addendum-2015)	No assay mentioned
1823	Sterile Water for Injections	No assay mentioned
1824	Stilboestrol	Visible spectroscopy
1825	Stilboestrol Tablets	Visible spectroscopy
1826	Streptokinase	Enzyme assay
1827	Streptokinase Injection	Enzyme assay
1828	Streptomycin Injection	Antibiotic assay
1829	Streptomycin Sulphate	Antibiotic assay
1830	Streptomycin Tablets	Antibiotic assay
1831	Strong Glutaraldehyde Solution	Acid-base titration
1832	Succinylcholine Chloride	Non-Aqueous titration, $HClO_4$
1833	Succinylcholine Injection	Acid-base titration
1834	Sucralose	HPLC
1835	Sucrose	No assay mentioned
1836	Sulphacetamide Eye Drops	Diazotisation titration (Nitrite titration)
1837	Sulphacetamide Sodium	Diazotisation titration (Nitrite titration)
1838	Sulphadiazine	Diazotisation titration (Nitrite titration)
1839	Sulphadiazine Tablets	Diazotisation titration (Nitrite titration)
1840	Sulphadoxine	Diazotisation titration (Nitrite titration)
1841	Sulphamethizole	Diazotisation titration (Nitrite titration)
1842	Sulphamethoxazole	Diazotisation titration (Nitrite titration)

Contd...

S. No	Title of Monograph	Assay Method Mentioned
1843	Sulpiride	Non-Aqueous titration, $HClO_4$
1844	Sulpiride Tablets	UV spectroscopy
1845	Sumatriptan	HPLC
1846	Sumatriptan Injection	HPLC
1847	Sumatriptan Succinate	HPLC
1848	Surgical Spirit	For methyl salicylate-UV spectroscopy; for diethyl phthalate-UV spectroscopy
1849	Tadalafil (Addendum-2015)	HPLC
1850	Tadalafil Tablets (Addendum-2015)	HPLC
1851	Talc	No assay mentioned
1852	Tamoxifen Citrate	Non-Aqueous titration, $HClO_4$
1853	Tamoxifen Tablets	UV spectroscopy
1854	Tamsulosin Hydrochloride	Non-Aqueous titration, $HClO_4$
1855	Tamsulosin Prolonged-release Capsules (Addendum-2015)	HPLC
1856	Tapentadol Hydrochloride	HPLC
1857	Tartaric Acid	Acid-base titration
1858	Tauroursodeoxycholic Acid	HPLC
1859	Teicoplanin	Antibiotic assay
1860	Telmisartan	HPLC
1861	Telmisartan Tablets	HPLC
1862	Temozolomide	HPLC
1863	Temozolomide Capsules	HPLC
1864	Tenofovir and Emtricitabine Tablets	HPLC
1865	Tenofovir Disoproxil Fumarate	HPLC
1866	Tenofovir Disoproxil Fumarate Tablets	HPLC
1867	Tenofovir Disoproxil Fumarate, Lamivudine and Efavirenz Tablets	HPLC
1868	Terazosin Hydrochloride	Acid-base titration

Contd...

S. No	Title of Monograph	Assay Method Mentioned
1869	Terazosin Tablets (Addendum-2015)	HPLC
1870	Terbutaline Inhalation	Visible spectroscopy
1871	Terbutaline Injection	Visible spectroscopy
1872	Terbutaline Sulphate	Non-Aqueous titration, $HClO_4$
1873	Terbutaline Tablets	Visible spectroscopy
1874	Testosterone Propionate	UV spectroscopy
1875	Testosterone Propionate Injection	UV spectroscopy
1876	Tetracycline	HPLC
1877	Tetracycline Capsules	HPLC
1878	Tetracycline Hydrochloride	HPLC
1879	Tetracycline Ointment	HPLC
1880	Theophylline	Acid-base titration
1881	Theophylline Injection	For theophylline-UV spectroscopy; for dextrose-Optical rotation
1882	Theophylline Prolonged-release Tablets	HPLC
1883	Thiabendazole	Non-Aqueous titration, $HClO_4$
1884	Thiabendazole Tablets	UV spectroscopy
1885	Thiacetazone	Gravimetry
1886	Thiacetazone and Isoniazid Tablets	For thiaacetazone-UV spectroscopy; for isoniazid-Oxidation-reduction titration (bromate titration-potentiometry)
1887	Thiamine Hydrochloride	Non-Aqueous titration, $HClO_4$
1888	Thiamine Injection	HPLC
1889	Thiamine Mononitrate	Non-Aqueous titration, $HClO_4$
1890	Thiamine Tablets	HPLC
1891	Thiocolchicoside	HPLC
1892	Thiocolchicoside Capsules	HPLC
1893	Thiomersal	Precipitation titration (Ammonium thiocyanate)
1894	Thiopentone Injection	For thiopentone-Non-Aqueous titration (Lithium methoxide); for Sodium-Acid-base titration

Contd...

S. No	Title of Monograph	Assay Method Mentioned
1895	Thiopentone Sodium	For thiopentone-Non-Aqueous titration (Lithium methoxide); for Sodium-Acid-base titration
1896	Thiotepa	Acid-base titration
1897	Thiotepa Injection	HPLC
1898	Thymol	Oxidation-reduction titration (Bromine titration)
1899	Thyroxine Sodium	HPLC
1900	Thyroxine Tablets	HPLC
1901	Tibolone (Addendum-2015)	Acid-base titration (terminal alkyne)
1902	Tibolone Tablets (Addendum-2015)	HPLC
1903	Ticarcillin and Clavulanic Acid Injection	HPLC
1904	Timolol Eye Drops	UV spectroscopy
1905	Timolol Maleate	Non-Aqueous titration, $HClO_4$
1906	Timolol Tablets	UV spectroscopy
1907	Tinidazole	Non-Aqueous titration, $HClO_4$
1908	Tinidazole Tablets	UV spectroscopy
1909	Tiotropium Bromide Monohydrate	HPLC
1910	Tiotropium Bromide Powder for Inhalation	HPLC
1911	Titanium Dioxide	Oxidation-reduction titration (Ceric)
1912	Tizanidine Hydrochloride	HPLC
1913	Tizanidine Tablets	HPLC
1914	Tobramycin	Antibiotic assay
1915	Tobramycin Injection	Antibiotic assay
1916	Tocopheryl Acetate	Oxidation-reduction titration (Ceric)
1917	Tofluprost	HPLC
1918	Tolazamide	Acid-base titration
1919	Tolazamide Tablets	Acid-base titration
1920	Tolbutamide	Acid-base titration
1921	Tolbutamide Tablets	Acid-base titration

Contd...

S. No	Title of Monograph	Assay Method Mentioned
1922	Tolnaftate	UV spectroscopy
1923	Tolnaftate Cream	UV spectroscopy
1924	Tolnaftate Gel	UV spectroscopy
1925	Tolnaftate Topical Powder	HPLC
1926	Tolnaftate Topical Solution	UV spectroscopy
1927	Tolterodine Tartarate	HPLC
1928	Tolterodine Tartrate Tablets (Addendum-2015)	HPLC
1929	Tolvaptan	HPLC
1930	Topiramate	HPLC
1931	Topiramate Tablets	HPLC
1932	Topotecan Hydrochloride	HPLC
1933	Topotecan Injection	HPLC
1934	Torsemide (Addendum-2015)	HPLC
1935	Torsemide Tablets (Addendum-2015)	HPLC
1936	Tramadol Capsules	HPLC
1937	Tramadol Hydrochloride	Non-Aqueous titration, $HClO_4$
1938	Trandolapril	HPLC
1939	Trandolapril Tablets	HPLC
1940	Tranexamic Acid	Non-Aqueous titration, $HClO_4$
1941	Tranexamic Acid Injection	Acid-base titration
1942	Tranexamin Acid Tablets	Non-Aqueous titration, $HClO_4$
1943	Tranilast	Acid-base titration
1944	Travoprost	HPLC
1945	Travoprost Eye Drops	HPLC
1946	Triamcinolone	UV spectroscopy
1947	Triamcinolone Acetonide	UV spectroscopy
1948	Triamcinolone Acetonide Injection	HPLC
1949	Triamcinolone Tablets	HPLC
1950	Triamterene	Non-Aqueous titration, $HClO_4$
1951	Triamterene Capsules	UV spectroscopy
1952	Tribasic Calcium Phosphate	Complexometric titration
1953	Tributyl Citrate	Gas Chromatography

Contd...

S. No	Title of Monograph	Assay Method Mentioned
1954	Trichloromonofluoromethane	Gas Chromatography
1955	Triclofos Oral Solution	Argentometry titration (Volhard method)
1956	Triclofos Sodium	For Chloride-Argentometry (Volhard's method); for triclofos sodium-Acid-base titration
1957	Triethyl Citrate	Acid-base titration
1958	Trifluoperazine Hydrochloride	Non-Aqueous titration, $HClO_4$
1959	Trifluoperazine Injection	UV spectroscopy
1960	Trifluoperazine Tablets	UV spectroscopy
1961	Triflupromazine Hydrochloride	Non-Aqueous titration, $HClO_4$
1962	Triflupromazine Injection	UV spectroscopy
1963	Triflupromazine Tablets	UV spectroscopy
1964	Trimetazidine Hydrochloride	Argentometry (potentiometry)
1965	Trimethobenzamide Hydrochloride	Non-Aqueous titration, $HClO_4$
1966	Trimethoprim	Non-Aqueous titration, $HClO_4$
1967	Trimethoprim and Sulphamethoxazole Oral Suspension	For trimethoprim-UV spectroscopy; for sulphamethoxazole-Visible spectroscopy
1968	Trimethoprim and Sulphamethoxazole Tablets	For trimethoprim-UV spectroscopy; for sulphamethoxazole-Diazotization (Nitrite titration)
1969	Trimethoprim Tablets	UV spectroscopy
1970	Triprolidine Hydrochloride	Non-Aqueous titration, $HClO_4$
1971	Triprolidine Tablets	UV spectroscopy
1972	Trisodium Edetate Concentrate for Injection	Complexometric titration
1973	Tropicamide	Non-Aqueous titration, $HClO_4$
1974	Tropicamide Eye Drops	UV spectroscopy
1975	Troxidone	Gas Chromatography
1976	Troxidone Capsules	Gas Chromatography

Contd...

S. No	Title of Monograph	Assay method mentioned
1977	Tubocurarine Chloride	UV spectroscopy
1978	Tubocurarine Injection	UV spectroscopy
1979	Tyrothricin	Antibiotic assay
1980	Udenafil	HPLC
1981	Ulipristal Acetate	HPLC
1982	Undecenoic acid	Acid-base titration
1983	Urea	Acid-base titration
1984	Urea Cream	Visible spectroscopy
1985	Urokinase	Enzyme Assay
1986	Ursodeoxycholic Acid	Acid-base titration
1987	Ursodeoxycholic Acid Tablets	HPLC
1988	Valproic Acid	Acid-base titration
1989	Valproic Acid Capsules	Gas Chromatography
1990	Valproic Acid Oral Solution	Gas Chromatography
1991	Valsartan	HPLC
1992	Valsartan and Hydrochlorothiazide Tablets	HPLC
1993	Valsartan Tablets	HPLC
1994	Vancomycin Capsules	Antibiotic assay
1995	Vancomycin Hydrochloride	Antibiotic assay
1996	Vancomycin Hydrochloride for Intravenous Infusion	Antibiotic assay
1997	Vancomycin Intravenous Infusion	Antibiotic assay
1998	Vancomycin Oral Solution	Antibiotic assay
1999	Vanillin	Acid-base titration
2000	Vasopressin	HPLC
2001	Vasopressin Injection	HPLC
2002	Vecuronium Bromide	Non-Aqueous titration, $HClO_4$
2003	Vecuronium Bromide Injection	HPLC
2004	Verapamil Hydrochloride	Non-Aqueous titration, $HClO_4$
2005	Verapamil Injection	UV spectroscopy
2006	Verapamil Tablets	UV spectroscopy

Contd…

S. No	Title of Monograph	Assay Method Mentioned
2007	Vinblastine Injection	UV spectroscopy
2008	Vinblastine Sulphate	HPLC
2009	Vincristine Injection	UV spectroscopy
2010	Vincristine Sulphate	HPLC
2011	Vinorelbine Injection	HPLC
2012	Vinorelbine Tartrate	HPLC
2013	Vitamin A Capsules	HPLC
2014	Vitamin A Concentrate Oil	UV spectroscopy
2015	Vitamin A Concentrate Powder	UV spectroscopy
2016	Vitamin A Paediatric Oral Solution	HPLC
2017	Vitamins A and D Capsules	For vitamin A-UV spectroscopy; for vitamin D-Column chromatography and visible spectroscopy
2018	Voglibose	Non-Aqueous titration, $HClO_4$
2019	Voglibose Dispersible Tablets	HPLC
2020	Voglibose Tablets	HPLC
2021	Voriconazole (Addendum-2015)	HPLC
2022	Voriconazole Tablets (Addendum-2015)	HPLC
2023	Warfarin Sodium	UV spectroscopy
2024	Warfarin Sodium Clathrate	UV spectroscopy
2025	Warfarin Tablets	UV spectroscopy
2026	Water for Injection	No assay mentioned
2027	Water for Injections in Bulk	No assay mentioned
2028	Water-Miscible Vitamin A Concentrate	UV spectroscopy
2029	White Beeswax	No assay mentioned
2030	White soft Paraffin	No assay mentioned
2031	Wool Fat	No assay mentioned
2032	Xanthan Gum	UV spectroscopy

Contd...

S. No	Title of Monograph	Assay Method Mentioned
2033	Xylometazoline Hydrochloride	Non-Aqueous titration, $HClO_4$
2034	Xylometazoline Nasal Drops	Visible spectroscopy
2035	Xylose	Visible spectroscopy
2036	Yellow Beeswax	No assay mentioned
2037	Yellow Soft Paraffin	No assay mentioned
2038	Zidovudine	HPLC
2039	Zidovudine Capsules	HPLC
2040	Zidovudine Injection	HPLC
2041	Zidovudine Oral Solution	HPLC
2042	Zidovudine Tablets	HPLC
2043	Zidovudine, Lamivudine and Nevirapine Tablets	HPLC
2044	Zinc Chloride	Complexometric titration
2045	Zinc Chloride Injection	Atomic absorption spectrometry
2046	Zinc Oxide	Complexometric titration
2047	Zinc Oxide and Salicylic Acid Paste	For salicylic acid-UV spectroscopy; for zinc oxide-Complexometry titration
2048	Zinc Oxide Cream	Complexometric titration
2049	Zinc Sterate	Complexometric titration
2050	Zinc Sulphate	Complexometric titration
2051	Zinc Sulphate Dispersible Tablets	Complexometric titration
2052	Zinc Sulphate Eye Drops	Complexometric titration
2053	Zinc Sulphate Monohydrate	Complexometric titration
2054	Zinc Sulphate Oral Solution	Complexometric titration
2055	Zinc Undecenoate	Complexometric titration
2056	Zinc Undecenoate Ointment	For zinc undecenoate-Complexometry titration; for free undecenoic acid-Acid-base titration
2057	Zoledronic Acid	HPLC

Contd...

S. No	Title of Monograph	Assay Method Mentioned
2058	Zoledronic Acid Injection	HPLC
2059	Zolmitriptan	HPLC
2060	Zolmitriptan Tablets	HPLC
2061	Zolpidem Tablets	HPLC
2062	Zolpidem Tartrate	Non-Aqueous titration, $HClO_4$
2063	Zonisamide	HPLC
2064	Zopiclone	Non-Aqueous titration, $HClO_4$
2065	Zopiclone Tablets	HPLC
2066	Zuclopenthixol Acetate	Non-Aqueous titration, $HClO_4$
2067	Zuclopenthixol Acetate Injection	HPLC

Question Bank for *viva-voce*

1. Define impurity?
2. What is a limit test?
3. Why limit tests are quantitative, semi-quantitative tests?
4. Why limit tests are called as comparative tests?
5. How can we predict the possible impurities of a drug substance?
6. What are the units for limit tests?
7. What should be the criteria in selection of Nessler's cylinders for performing limit tests?
8. What is opalescence?
9. What is turbidity?
10. What are the sources for chloride impurities imparting into test substance?
11. Why in limit test for chlorides, dilute nitric acid is used?
12. What is the standard impurity used in limit test for chlorides?
13. What is the principle involved in limit test for chlorides?
14. What is the difference between limit test for chlorides when compared to limit test for sulphates, heavy metals and iron?
15. What are the sources for sulphate impurities imparting into test substance?
16. Why dilute acetic acid or dilute hydrochloric acid used in limit test for sulphates?
17. What is the difference in limit test for sulphates among different Indian pharmacopoeia?
18. What is the purpose of intentional addition of sulphate impurity in both standard and test Nessler cylinder in limit test for sulphates.
19. What is the role of ethyl alcohol in limit test for sulphates.
20. What are the sources for iron impurities imparting into test substance?

21. Which form of iron (i.e., ferric or ferrous) gives observation in limit test for iron?

22. What are the roles of thioglycollic acid in limit test for iron?

23. What are the roles of citric acid in limit test for iron?

24. What is the role of ammonia in limit test for iron?

25. What are the sources for heavy metals imparting into test substance?

26. What are the different heavy metals?

27. Why lead even though heavy metal, an exclusive limit test for lead being included in various pharmacopoeias?

28. What is the role of pH in limit test for heavy metals?

29. What are the different methods of limit test for heavy metals in Indian pharmacopoeia?

30. What are the sources for arsenic impurities imparting into test substance?

31. Describe the apparatus used in limit test for arsenic?

32. What are the two forms of arsenic ions?

33. To what form arsenic ions are converted into on addition of hydrochloric acid in limit test for arsenic?

34. How are arsenic and arsenous acids converted to arsine gas?

35. What is the reaction of arsine with mercuric chloride?

36. What is the role of zinc and hydrochloric acid in limit test for arsenic?

37. What is the role of lead acetate cotton/paper in limit test for arsenic?

38. What is the role of stannated hydrochloric acid (includes $SnCl_2$ and HCl) in limit test for arsenic?

39. What is the purpose of side hold in the design of the apparatus of limit test for arsenic?

40. What is the role of potassium iodide in limit test for arsenic?

41. Why the reagent used in limit test for arsenic suffixed with AsT?

42. What is the other name for limit test for arsenic?

43. What are the sources for lead impurities imparting into test substance?

44. What is the colour of dithizone in chloroform?

45. What is the colour of lead dithizone complex in chloroform?

46. What is the role of ammonium citrate, hydroxylamine hydrochloride and potassium cyanide in limit test for lead?

47. Why the solution is made alkaline before addition of potassium cyanide in limit test for lead?

48. What is the difference between dithizone extract solution and dithizone standard solution?

49. What are the standard impurities in limit test for sulphates, iron, heavy metals, arsenic and lead?

50. Why dilute reagents are used in limit tests?

51. What are the different reactions in limit test for chlorides, sulphates, iron, heavy metals, arsenic and lead?

52. What are the modifications necessary if limit test has to be performed for a coloured substance (especially limit test for chlorides, sulphates, iron, heavy metals)?

53. What are the modifications necessary if limit test has to be performed for a water insoluble substance?

54. Explain the principle involved in limit test?

55. Explain the specific principle involved in limit test for chlorides, sulphates, heavy metals, iron, lead and arsenic?

56. What are the problems aroused when impurity in drug substance is beyond the limits?

57. Chlorides are present in the body. What happens if chloride impurities are present in the drug substance?

58. Why less specific reagents are used in limit tests?

59. What is the role of nitric acid in limit test for lead?

60. Define assay?

61. Compare estimation with an assay?

62. What are the different types of assays or estimations?

63. What is redox titration?

64. What is acid-base titration?

65. What is argentometric titration?

66. What is precipitation titration?

67. What is complexometric titration?

68. What is non-aqueous titration?

69. Give examples of different indicators?

70. What type of compounds are assayed by non-aqueous titration?

71. What happens if water is present in non-aqueous titration?

72. Give examples for different types of assays?

73. What are the different types of precipitation titrations?

74. What are the different methods of spectrometric assays or estimations?